Praise f

"Systems thinking has been around for a long time. But thoughtful application of its insights has been few and far between—especially in institutions where they have been desperately needed. Dr. Slakey has just changed all that by successfully integrating his innovative research and vast experience as an accomplished surgeon. The result is a truly unique and eye-opening guide that can finally put us on the right path to effective management of our incredibly complex healthcare system."

—Gökçe Sargut, PhD. Associate Professor of Business, Governors State University

"*The Process Manifesto* illuminates much of what healthcare currently lacks and provides an evidence-based approach to improvement. Dr. Slakey has the vision to apply reliability science—much of which lies outside the medical community's traditional education and operational experience—to the constantly changing healthcare delivery model. The book should be required reading for any healthcare professional. Patients, too, would benefit from seeing, understanding, and demanding more from our healthcare systems."

—K. Scott Griffith, author of *The Leader's Guide to Managing Risk: A Proven Method to Build Resilience and Reliability*

"Dr. Slakey has served patients, caregivers and worked with teams in the most critical situations. The Ten Core Principles for Complex System Process Management in Healthcare are realistic and actionable. His advocacy for strong process allows our most powerful gifts to be set free: the front line caregivers and patients. Let's go! "

—Katie Kaney, DRPH, MBA, FACHE, Author of *BOTH/AND*

"As a career technology executive, I've found myself interested in how proven approaches to process improvement could be applied to the complex and often mysterious healthcare system. Dr. Slakey's insightful book offers a comprehensive roadmap to do just that. Drawing on a real-world approach, it provides practical strategies to design processes to enhance efficiency ensuring the core mission of patient care quality and outcomes remains center. With real-world case studies and actionable advice, it equips healthcare professionals and senior leaders with the tools needed to drive meaningful improvements. Whether you're a practitioner, administrator, or executive in the healthcare industry, this book is an invaluable resource for achieving operational excellence and delivering better patient outcomes—using approaches that have proven themselves in countless other industries. It's time for healthcare to move forward."

—Frank Bien, ex-CEO Looker

"Dr Slakey has deftly incorporated great minds from all disciplines into the optimization of healthcare delivery with the needs of the patient always coming first. I have been privileged to work in stellar medical platforms across the world. None greater than what Dr Slakey has created. Always strong work."

—Pam Gillette, MPH, RN, FACHE

"As someone who has surveyed hundreds of hospitals large and small as part of a healthcare accreditation organization (DNV), Douglas Slakey, MD MPH, has written a must-read primer for anyone who has ever tried to impact change in large, complex organizations. The book reads as a thoughtful, step-by-step guide to help organizations to understand the dynamics of the process-driven approach to positively impact quality, safety, communication, costs, and patient-centric outcomes. *The Process Manifesto* is written in a way that is easy to understand with real-life examples and will surely be an invaluable tool for those people who are charged with effectuating meaningful and lasting process improvement in complex organizations."

—Thomas J. Quinn, MPA, LPC, DNV Healthcare
Accreditation Services

"Dr. Slakey is a compassionate advocate of multi-disciplinary teams for patients' long-term health and quality of life while diligently working towards improving the healthcare system for all. As Dr. Slakey's longtime patient, I prayerfully suggest doctors, nurses, and interns of all specialties to read, retain, and apply his book in their practice as well as with their patients."

—Kathy Burr, cancer survivor

THE
PROCESS
MANIFESTO

THE
PROCESS
MANIFESTO

**Improving
Healthcare
in a
Complex
World**

DOUGLAS SLAKEY, MD, MPH

A PROCESS HEALTH CONSULTING LLC BOOK
Processhealthconsulting.com

ISBN (paperback): 979-8-9892576-0-7
ISBN (ebook): 979-8-9892576-1-4

Printed in the United States of America

Book design and production by www.AuthorSuccess.com

Library of Congress Control Number: 2023920144

This work depicts actual events in the life of the author as truthfully as recollection permits. While all persons within are actual individuals, names and identifying characteristics have been changed to respect their privacy.

To my wife Jeanette and my children Christina, Lauren, and Austin,
who continuously support me in my search for answers
and who inspire me to do my best.

CONTENTS

FOREWORD

I have known Doug Slakey, M.D. for over twenty years. We first met when I was the chief of neurosurgery at Memorial Hospital, an indigent hospital on the Gulf Coast of Mississippi. I have previously been a professor of neurosurgery at Stanford University and had taken a sabbatical initially to do an entrepreneurial activity, but also to consult on occasion for hospitals wishing to develop neuroscience/orthopedic centers of excellence. After visiting the hospital, I was moved by the fact that there was no credible neurosurgery, no neurology, no consistent orthopedic surgery, and no integrated plan of how to improve the situation. The hospital goal was focused on these physicians covering the emergency room, with no plan beyond.

This strategy resulted in applicants for the various positions often having had issues related to prior drug and alcohol abuse, personality issues that resulted in them being fired from prior positions, and often, recent divorces. After presenting a plan to the hospital board that focused on finding quality physicians to build an integrated center of excellence versus simply advertising for bodies to cover the emergency room, they voted unanimously to move forward, recognizing it would take a minimum of three years and several million dollars. The caveat was that they wanted me to accept the position as the director of this nascent program.

After long discussion with my wife, I accepted the position and left Stanford. Fortunately, not only did my prior experience at Stanford give me insights into program development, but my years in private practice also gave me significant insights, as well. And so it began. Over the period I was there, we not only filled the slots, but filled them with highly qualified applicants. Additionally, we built an integrated team that was co-located in the same offices and created a neuro ICU and a dedicated floor for neurosurgery, neurology, and orthopedic patients. We also created the first brain injury, stroke, and trauma rehabilitation facility and the first Stroke Center Certification in the state.

The other great aspect was that I was less than an hour away from Tulane Medical School, which I had attended and was on the Board of Governors. As a result, I could interact and get advice and insights from colleagues from a variety of specialties and with a variety of experiences. It was from these experiences that Doug and I became friends, as he was the chief of surgery at Tulane at the time. What further strengthened our relationship was Hurricane Katrina. We had many conversations regarding how to rebuild healthcare in New Orleans, especially focusing on patient-centric care and processes while also addressing the barriers that prevent this, which is often social and cultural.

While I stayed in Mississippi for two years after Hurricane Katrina, my wife and child moved back to California. Ultimately, while I very much enjoyed the professional aspects of my work there, it was untenable to remain, and I decided to return to Stanford. But in many ways, the work there had a huge impact and further strengthened my resolve regarding the importance of compassion in all areas of one's life, especially for healthcare workers, as so often the demands on us are antithetical to the needs of our patients. This results in a sense of moral injury for many. During this time, Doug and I continued to communicate regarding the need for examining the processes in healthcare that so often prevent us from doing our jobs, whether that be as physicians, nurses, or healthcare workers.

In the meantime, I founded a center at Stanford (The Center for Compassion and Altruism Research and Education) focused on understanding the neuroscience of compassion and how it is integral to human flourishing. Extraordinarily, His Holiness the Dalai Lama became our founding benefactor, and I ultimately became the chairman of the Dalai Lama Foundation. Because of my friendship and admiration of Doug, I invited him to an event I was hosting at Stanford with His Holiness and made an introduction. In many ways, it was this introduction that crystalized Doug's desire to examine the complexity that is modern healthcare, with often misaligned incentives and a focus on finances, often to the detriment of patient care. Doug shared with me that following his visit to Stanford and meeting the Dalai Lama and reading his books, it realigned him with his moral compass and made him realize that as a physician leader he could move the needle, ultimately receiving numerous grants which allowed him to gain further insights and knowledge that led him to provide education, training, and coaching to caregiver teams with the goal of empowering them to increase access and provide care to more of the community they served, much of which was based on the principles he learned during and after Hurricane Katrina.

What I hadn't realized was that following the publication of my *New York Times* and international bestselling memoir, *Into the Magic Shop: A Neurosurgeon's Quest to Discover the Mysteries of the Brain and the Secrets of the Heart*, Doug read it, and this further impacted his journey to write the volume that is in your hand. According to Doug, my book taught him patience, perspective, and the fundamental importance of the doctor-patient relationship, and just as importantly, the healthcare-system relationship. He realized that due to the complexity of healthcare, especially concerning the uniqueness of each of us as individuals, we cannot reduce our interactions and decisions to an overly standardized, linear approach. Instead, we must embrace complexity and provide ways to enhance our and the patient's experience. Fundamentally, he embraced compassion, which is at the core of human relationships.

He summarized the three main principles of the *Process Manifesto*: Process, Intention, and Opening the Heart.

In regard to *Process*, Doug has defined it as responding to flow disruptions and how one must empower the individual to be the most effective and efficient in responding to the need, specifically that of the patient. It is the leaders and all who work within healthcare systems that must consider their processes regarding accepting complexity, uniqueness of the individual, mutual respect, and compassion. This includes:

1. Optimizing process to empower the individual to be most effective and efficient in responding to need (i.e., patient need).

2. Recognizing and managing process flow disruptions to maximize the patient experience.

Additionally, one must clarify one's *Intention* if one is to create sustainable change in oneself or within an organization, which includes:

1. Ensuring that patient-centric care and outcomes are the ultimate measures of success.

2. Empowering people by implementing processes that optimize human performance and thriving.

3. Dedication to implementing highly reliable processes that align resources with individual patient need.

And lastly, *Opening One's Heart*, which oftentimes is the most difficult as such terms are not typically used within the normal nomenclature of healthcare. This includes:

1. Effectively managing complexity by allowing healthcare professionals to align the reasons for their work (providing care) and the existing incentives concerning the process.

2. Realizing that human health (care) is a right and necessary to relieve suffering. This realization should influence those involved (especially leaders responsible for the processes by which care is delivered) to ensure that the system/processes are providing care that is consistent with the ultimate objective of helping others and relieving suffering.

To me, what is the most powerful in the entire text is what Doug calls the *Ten Core Principles for Complex System Process Management in Healthcare*, which are:

1. Patient-centric quality outcomes are the primary measure of success.

   a. Focus on the outcome of the process, not the process itself.

2. Embrace complexity.

   a. Design responsive and adaptable processes to manage the unexpected.

   b. Avoid trying to reduce patient care to a linear, assembly-line process.

3. Create and empower teams of teams

a. Give them the tools they need to succeed.

b. Reduce the negative impact of silos, especially at the point of care.

c. Accountability becomes "What do you need for success?" instead of "What went wrong?"

4. Utilize evidence-based practice

a. Establish patient-centered care guidelines and associated processes.

b. Patient-centered care processes provide a structured approach to patient treatment plans, helping to reduce variability in care.

5. Align resources and information at the point of care to optimize team performance.

6. Make education and training a priority

a. Providing health workers with ongoing training and resources will increase their understanding of patient care needs, leading to more informed decisions about patient treatment processes.

b. Include situational awareness training.

7. Provide actionable, accurate information

a. Utilizing data analytics allows healthcare providers to make the best patient care decisions based on a comprehensive understanding of the patient.

8. Leverage technology

   a. Where appropriate, automate and streamline aspects of patient care processes to improve accuracy by removing potential human error from critical decision-making steps.

9. Create an environment where everyone contributes to high-quality patient care

   a. Reward innovation and transformative change.

   b. Optimize processes by understanding how each step contributes to patient outcomes.

10. Be compassionate

Complexity in healthcare imposes challenges, but there are ways it can be managed, though not controlled. Increasing our ability to improve healthcare in a complex world is a journey, not a destination. What lights the path of this journey is seeing the world through the lens of compassion.

I am honored to have shared a bit of this journey with Doug and believe that what is contained in this "Manifesto" has the potential to have a huge impact on healthcare, but most importantly on our patients and on ourselves.

James R Doty, MD, Adjunct Professor, Stanford University School of Medicine and author of *Into the Magic Shop: A Neurosurgeon's Quest to Discover the Mysteries of the Brain and the Secrets of the Heart.*

PROLOGUE

I was sitting with the chair of surgery and the hospital CEO, and neither was very happy. It was Friday, August 26, 2005, and I, as the director of the abdominal transplant program, had informed the United Network for Organ Sharing (UNOS) that we would not be accepting organs for transplantation until Hurricane Katrina passed. Katrina had rapidly intensified to a Category 5 storm over the warm Gulf waters. No one was certain where Katrina would make landfall, but New Orleans was directly in the projected path.

The room was tense, and I explained my concern about patient safety. Our center had performed over 200 liver, kidney, and pancreas transplants during the previous twelve months. We were very busy as a team, but volume was not our top priority. The transplant team was committed to individualized patient care and optimizing outcomes. Ensuring that patients received safe, reliable, high-quality care was our priority. The transplant team was very concerned that patients would suffer and might even die if Katrina brought the devastation to New Orleans that some predicted.

My experience as an offshore sailor taught me to respect the power of nature. The intensity and size of Katrina scared me. I imagined what it would be like to care for immunosuppressed transplant patients without electricity, air conditioning, lights, and a shortage of life-saving medications. The full transplant team would not be present as people evacuated. The team members were looking for leadership and permission to protect our patients and care for their families. The hospital executives were planning to shelter in place with minimal staffing.

I said, "I made the decision because of the unpredictability of the storm. If we have patients in the hospital and we are without electricity, water, air conditioning, and critical medications, people will die. What if we need blood and the blood bank is closed? If patients die, you will blame me and the team."

"You are completely overreacting. You have no right to close the program or send patients elsewhere," they said almost in unison. "What are you going to do with the patients?"

"I am the program director, so I have an ethical and regulatory responsibility. The transplant team has determined that we can send most of the in-patients home, and if we cancel our elective cases, we will have only one patient remaining in the hospital. We have contacted other centers out of the storm's path that can take patients as needed. Our processes allow us to refer patients waiting for a transplant to other centers if that becomes necessary."

"We certainly do not want to lose that business."

"No," I replied. "They are our patients, and we would only transfer them to other centers if it was the worst-case scenario."

I walked back to the transplant offices feeling frustrated after that exchange. My partner asked how the meeting went.

"I was told I was overreacting and had no right to close the transplant program. They asked me how I could do something so dramatic while other surgeons continued with full schedules as though it was a normal day."

My partner said, "That's ridiculous. Patient and staff safety should be the priority. Do you know that Dr. Smith (not his real name) is doing an elective gastric bypass on a 520-pound person right now?"

"Well, they clearly think it is just fine to operate on patients without concern about something like a hurricane."

Katrina made landfall on August 29. In the transplant unit, only one patient remained in the hospital; the others were safely out of Katrina's path. The gastric bypass patient was on a ventilator. As the hurricane passed and the winds subsided, there was initial euphoria—the hospital, patients, and staff were fine, and there did not seem to be too much damage to the city. Then the water began to rise.

The levy system failed, and 80 percent of New Orleans was underwater. People suffered. The patients and staff in the hospital lived in unimaginable conditions suffering from heat and humidity, lack of running water, shortages of supplies, and no relief. The toilets did not work, and people were forced to use plastic bags. Cellphones stopped working. Gunshots were regularly heard. No one could come or go due to the flooded streets. Days and nights passed by, slowly and painfully. When would the suffering end? In some hospitals, people began dying.

All the patients and staff in our hospital were eventually evacuated by helicopter a week after the storm. It was truly a miracle. Other hospitals were not as fortunate, and in the end, over 200 hospitalized patients were to die.

The 520-pound gastric bypass patient and others who could not walk had to be carried down several flights of stairs in pitch darkness, then through a parking lot and up several ramps to the top floor where they could be placed into helicopters and flown to safety. The heroism of the staff and the support of the administration were undeniable.

Even before the flood waters fully receded, another physician and I collected transplant patient records from our office on the seventeenth floor. We carried boxes down pitch-black stairwells using headlamps and filled our SUVs. Our patients were scattered across three states. We set up temporary clinics, drove endless miles, ate ready-to-eat meals provided by the national guard, slept on couches of generous people we barely knew, and reconnected with patients. A pharmaceutical company generously flew in a chartered plane with precious immunosuppressive drugs our transplant patients needed. None of our patients lost their transplanted organs.

Recovery began. The hospital re-opened in February 2006—six months after Katrina devastated New Orleans. On Valentine's Day, we did our first transplant since the storm, a living donor transplant from a husband to his wife. For the transplant team this was a celebration of resilience.

The unpredictable course of Katrina and the unexpected failure of the levy system made us aware that there are things we cannot control. As Katrina approached, the variability of the hospital and health system leadership decisions revealed layers of complexity. First, there were competing agendas and perspectives. My team's decision to close the transplant program did not align with the administrative decision to continue elective cases until the last minute. If the levies had not failed, my decision would have been viewed by some as the wrong decision. In fact, some continued questioning my decision to close the transplant program and send the hospitalized transplant patients to safety before Katrina.

The existing process was to keep going as usual and "shelter in place" until the danger had passed. I began to consider how we should balance risk with patient safety in a rational way. Continuing elective surgery and keeping so many patients in the hospital produced an unnecessary avoidable risk. Still, the processes and policies in many ways encouraged and rewarded increased risk. Is putting fellow human beings, including the most vulnerable, at increased risk the right thing to do?

What motivated the surgeons who had kept operating on elective patients as the storm made landfall? Often surgeons are compared to Top Gun pilots, and a degree of hubris and risk-taking is seen as a badge of honor. Hadn't they succeeded by evacuating the hospital despite tremendous adversity and, fortunately, in our case, without loss of life? Was the pressure to keep hospital beds full and the operating rooms busy and making money affecting judgment? Were the decisions heroic or something else?

This became a turning point for me and my career. Was it better to accept more risk than was necessary? Would a ship captain purposefully steer into a Category 5 hurricane when they could avoid it? Would an airline pilot responsible for 200 passengers (the number of patients our hospital had) think their experience would ensure a safe and reliable outcome in the face of 170-mile-an-hour winds? Would subjecting airline passengers to unnecessary risk be tolerated?

Our healthcare system should be guided by high-reliability principles prioritizing safety and quality. Hurricane Katrina exposed a paradox where a professed commitment to safety contrasted with a willingness to accept more risk than was necessary. Our healthcare system is complex because there are so many aspects to it, many having competing misaligned incentives. The outcome measures that define success are sometimes different depending upon perspective. Keeping a hospital busy and full may not align with preventative healthcare goals of keeping patients out of the hospital.

The system's complexity is inseparable from unpredictability and never fully knowable or controllable. There had to be a way to resolve these differences and re-prioritize how we provided care. I realized the processes needed to be improved so that outcomes like patient-centric care, quality, reliability, and value became prioritized. The excessive cost of healthcare can be better managed if processes are more efficient and effective, reducing waste. Incentives had to become aligned.

I asked, "If we cannot control our complex healthcare world, how can we manage it more effectively, ensuring a patient-centric approach and providing value?"

The answer is by optimizing processes—aligning incentives and resources so that healthcare teams can work most effectively when and where they are caring for patients.

By optimizing processes, we can empower the healthcare team to do the right thing for the right patient at the right time.[1]

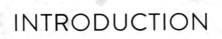

INTRODUCTION

"For every complex problem,
there is an answer that is clear, simple, and wrong."
H.L. MENCKEN

At some point in our lives, each of us will be a patient and, at some point, each of us a caregiver. As people, we are together, inseparable from the healthcare system. Whenever we talk about the healthcare system, we are talking about people, no matter if our focus is on patients or providers or the administrators who do their best to make sense of complicated economic realities.

Ultimately, our efforts must be guided by compassion, not only to make sense of our efforts to improve the care we provide but also to understand the challenges of all working each day doing their best to improve patients's lives and reduce suffering.

○ ○ ○

Recently I read a LinkedIn® post written by a well-known physician who is the president of a large medical group. He was sharing his experience as a roundtable member discussing the large number of hospital and health system mergers and acquisitions occurring nationwide. The conclusion was that the mergers, some creating huge organizations, were driven by "finances and workforce challenges." These challenges are real, driven by many factors, including the effects of the Covid pandemic. Healthcare finances affect all of us. The United States's healthcare spending is approaching 17 percent of GDP, far exceeding any other Western country, with healthcare outcomes not consistently better than those of other nations and, by some measures, worse.[2]

I read the post with interest, but, almost like a Greek tragedy, I was left unsettled by the reasons supporting the mergers. I thought that if the healthcare system was truly delivering on its promises to the population, the roundtable participants should have concluded that the mergers were being driven by "the need to improve the ability to deliver highly reliable, safe, and effective patient care."

○ ○ ○

Patient care, and the patient experience, occur in a complex system. Process flow describes the efficiency and reliability of events within that system and the fundamental process functions. Too often, health systems have attempted to reduce processes to a linear, highly predictable, and structured construct. This reductionist approach does not fully appreciate the complexity of caring for individual patients. Further, the inevitable unpredictability and variation of health care and patient need cannot be accommodated safely when provider teams are overly restricted and unable to adapt to circumstances that arise during patient care.

Appreciating and understanding processes in a complex environment is essential for healthcare systems to function with the highest reliability. Complex systems have multiple separate but interdependent components with multiple stakeholders involved.

A challenge exists because of independent units operating within the healthcare system with different budgets, different leadership, and performance metrics that are frequently incompatible. However, there is no question that they are completely interdependent where patient care is concerned. To optimize process flow during patient care, all professional units that provide, pay for, and support patient care must be tightly coupled. Overly rigid, linear process management can prevent or inhibit the ability of professionals to respond to process flow disruptions, especially at the point of patient care delivery.

> *Linear systems might be great for manufacturing cars on an assembly line, but we are not making cars; our healthcare system is caring for people. Patients are individuals that have unique histories and needs.*

We spend large amounts of money and time training professionals to be experts and able to react to unexpected situations. We train them to prevent or intercede to reduce the potential for process flow disruptions that may result in adverse events. Unfortunately, the system can *(and does)* often impose rigid standards that prevent optimal process flow. This adversely impacts patient care and the patient experience.

Ultimately, to improve the reliability of patient care and ensure greater safety and value in care delivery, everyone working within the health system must acknowledge that patient care occurs within a complex environment that cannot be reduced to an overly rigid linear system model. The health care system must manage complexity to allow its professionals to have the training, information, and resources necessary to respond appropriately to optimize process flow and provide optimal patient care.

I have committed myself to understanding the impact of complexity on our healthcare system. I have thought about and asked many experts, "How can we better manage complexity by creating processes prioritizing patient-centric outcomes, safety, reliability, and quality?"

My research and work have always focused on putting patient outcomes first. I established and partnered with diverse teams to create process improvement strategies to increase quality and reliability and to manage resources more effectively to control cost. My work has demonstrated improved patient access, better outcomes, reduced costs, and improved patient and healthcare team satisfaction.

My quest for optimizing processes in healthcare has taken me around the world, where I have been fortunate to work closely with many healthcare experts and teams. I have partnered with high-reliability and safety experts in medicine and other industries such as aerospace, transportation, and energy. As I traveled the world, I realized that universally people were looking for ways to become more effective and efficient in caring for patients. I increasingly understood that there were elements of process improvement that healthcare teams everywhere could use to be more effective and efficient.

I have come to realize that optimizing processes means improving human performance.

The mission of this book is to provide a foundational perspective that enables people working in healthcare to accomplish three objectives:

1. Ensuring that patient-centric care and outcomes are the ultimate measures of success.

2. Empowering people by implementing processes that optimize human performance.

3. Dedication to implementing highly reliable processes that align resources with individual patient need.

This book supports a call to action that focuses on improving processes within healthcare systems to improve healthcare and patient outcomes. It emphasizes the importance of planning and flexibility when managing processes and how processes must align with patient-centric goals. Leadership's commitment to optimizing process flow and supporting those who make it work ensures the best opportunity for quality, safety, and reliability, along with accessibility and affordability.

The Process Manifesto provides readers with an understanding of how to create and manage effective processes by applying complex system theory.

Reading *The Process Manifesto* provides insight into improving existing processes to serve patients better and achieve desired outcomes. Readers will learn how to create efficient workflows, develop strategies for change management, and understand the importance of collaboration between different departments to ensure the successful implementation of processes. *The Process Manifesto* is a resource for anyone looking to improve their healthcare system by focusing on improving processes.

Empowering healthcare providers to do the right thing for the right patient at the right time cannot be overstated.

Healthcare providers are on the front lines of providing care and must have the knowledge and skills to make informed decisions about each patient's care. Empowerment is essential to this process. Complexity imposes demands upon both providers and patients. The processes within a complex environment are inconsistent and subject to unexpected patterns. Optimizing human performance within a complex environment requires the ability to react to situational realities as they exist and as they arise. Rigid, overly standardized processes and protocols cannot adapt rapidly enough to be reliable.

Improving healthcare processes in a complex environment is about empowering and enabling people to provide healthcare to people (as patients) that is the right care at the right time. Optimal processes create an environment where people at all levels thrive, including employee and patient satisfaction.

Supporting administrators and managers is an important goal of *The Process Manifesto*. Through the process of understanding complex system theory and then designing and implementing processes that more effectively manage complexity, leadership can be freed to concentrate efforts on strategy, lessening the struggle of endlessly putting out fires.

> *Moving from putting out fires to preventing them is foundational to process optimization.*

Leaders, no matter where within the healthcare system, they are, can apply the principles of complex system management to optimize the performance of processes within their sphere of influence. I have created and helped teams in the United States and around the world apply my ten core principles for managing patient care within the complex health system environment.

The 10 Core Principles for Complex System Process Management in Healthcare

1. Patient-centric quality outcomes are the primary measure of success.

    a. Focus on the outcome of the process, not the process itself.

2. Embrace complexity.

   a. Design responsive and adaptable processes to manage the unexpected.

   b. Avoid trying to reduce patient care to a linear, assembly-line process.

3. Create and empower teams of teams.

   a. Give them the tools they need to succeed.

   b. Reduce the negative impact of silos (departments that function independently), especially at the point of care delivery.

   c. Accountability becomes asking "what do you need for success?" instead of "what went wrong?"

4. Utilize evidence-based practices.

   a. Establish patient-centered care guidelines and associated processes.

   b. Patient-centered care processes provide a structured approach to patient treatment plans, helping to reduce variability in care.

5. Align resources and information at the point of care to optimize team performance.

6. Make education and training a priority.

   a. Providing health workers with ongoing training and resources will increase their understanding of patient care needs, leading to more informed decisions about patient treatment processes.

   b. Include situational awareness training.

7. Provide actionable, accurate information.

    a. Utilizing data analytics allows healthcare providers to make the best patient care decisions based on a comprehensive understanding of the patient.

8. Leverage technology.

    a. Where appropriate, automate and streamline aspects of patient care processes to improve accuracy by removing potential human error from critical decision-making steps.

9. Create an environment where everyone contributes to high-quality patient care.

    a. Reward innovation and transformative change.

    b. Optimize processes by understanding how each step contributes to patient outcomes.

10. Be compassionate.

Complexity in healthcare imposes challenges, but there are ways it can be managed, though not controlled. Increasing our ability to improve healthcare in a complex world is a journey, not a destination.

CHAPTER 1

THRIVING IN COMPLEXITY

"Eighty-five percent of the reasons for failure are deficiencies
in the systems and process rather than the employee.
The role of management is to change the process rather
than badgering individuals to do better."

W. EDWARDS DEMING,
IN *WHAT WOULD DEMING DO?* BY NILES PFLAEGING, ED.

Every patient knows first-hand that healthcare is complex. This becomes personal for each of us when faced with being *the patient*. This is a universal truth around the world. No matter where we live, how we pay for healthcare, or our familiarity with the system's nuances, every patient has a story of being frustrated as they go through their healthcare journey.

A fifty-nine-year-old woman, we will call her "Sally," recently decided to live out her dream and move to a beautiful mountain community. She had a career in healthcare administration. Her family was sophisticated medically, including having a daughter who is a surgical oncologist.

Sally got settled in her new home and made an appointment for her annual medical exam. Not unexpectedly, the primary care doctor could not see her as a new patient for three months. She asked the office if they would also schedule an annual mammogram in the meantime.

The mammogram was easily scheduled for a week later. After the mammogram, Sally received a call telling her they needed to do an ultrasound and additional studies. When comparing the new test with her past mammograms, some new microcalcifications were seen on the right side. The local cancer center's radiologist suggested that she have a biopsy. A stereotactic biopsy was done, and Sally was told to expect the results within five days. Sally told the radiologist and the cancer center nurse that she was leaving town for two weeks, so a phone call would be best.

Five days went by, then six days, and no call from the cancer center. Sally was becoming anxious, worried that she must have something serious.

On the seventh day, a primary care office staff member called. Remember, this was the office of a physician that Sally had never been to. The physician's office left a voice message stating that she needed to come in urgently that afternoon to meet with Dr. Dorby to discuss her biopsy results. This was a very foreboding message and Sally's worry increased. Sally called the office back and told the nurse that she was out of town, so she could not come in. She asked what the pathology result was. The office staff said they could not read anything over the phone because of HIPPA. Sally replied that if they could not tell her over the phone, would they please release the results into the EPIC medical record so she could read it?

The nurse said she could not release the results to EPIC without Dr. Dorby's approval. Sally asked if Dr. Dorby would please call her. A few hours later, not hearing anything, Sally called Dr. Dorby's office again. The nurse said she spoke to Dr. Dorby and that Sally had to come in to discuss the pathology results. By that time, she was more upset and, fearing the worst, wanted an answer. Sally reminded the nurse that she was out of town for two weeks, so making an in-person office visit was impossible. She reminded them that her daughter was a surgical oncologist and could help explain the results. Sally wanted to know so she could make plans and arrange treatment. Sally was imagining the worst case scenario, that she had a terrible result and was going to die.

The nurse said there was nothing she could do. Sally asked the office manager to call her, and the nurse said she would leave a message.

Sally then called the cancer center nurse navigator who had helped arrange the biopsy. Sally asked if she could release the pathology. The nurse navigator said she could not do that, and suggested Sally call the radiology department.

Sally called the radiology department. They said they did have the pathology results but could not tell Sally what those results were. They suggested calling the pathology office.

By this time, Sally was really going down the proverbial rabbit hole—she interpreted the lack of anyone giving her the results as a certain death sentence. She started thinking about which children would receive her jewelry, art, and the Mini Cooper! Worse yet, her son's wedding was four weeks away—how was that going to work now?

The pathology office was friendly and understanding but said they could do nothing; their processes and protocols did not allow them to give patients their results.

Sally was anxious, concerned, and frustrated all at the same time. The system was not working. The results, which were rightfully hers, were in reality—from a practical perspective—not hers. The results of her biopsy belonged to the health system, not Sally.

How could this be considered patient-centric? Who was in control? Not Sally.

The following morning Dr. Dorby's office manager called. Sally again explained that she was out of town and that she was anxious about the results and just wanted them released so that she could read the pathology on the patient portal.

The office manager said, "Giving the results over the phone or putting them into EPIC is impossible. You need to respect the doctor's judgment and wishes and make an appointment to come in to the office. If that is two weeks from now, that is just how it must be."

With tears streaming down her face resulting from emotions including frustration and anger, Sally responded, "What about my feelings as a patient? They are my results, and I want them now. This is not fair to me."

The office manager sharply and without compassion said, "I will let Dr. Dorby know and see if she will call you."

After taking a deep breath and composing herself, Sally called the cancer center again and spoke to the nurse navigator. She explained that she was upset, very concerned, and just wanted to know the biopsy results to start planning the next steps. The nurse was sympathetic and, after a few additional hours, was able to get a radiologist to call and read the pathology report to her.

Fortunately, the diagnosis was in-situ, early-stage cancer. Sally could finally begin to plan a treatment path and get the care she needed to treat her cancer.

Processes that are Not Patient-Centric

In managing Sally's biopsy, everyone followed a protocol or process that was too rigid and inflexible to respond to her as an individual. No one did anything wrong, but the system did not work and created avoidable mental trauma. The ability to respond to Sally compassionately was impossible due to the existing processes. Everyone within the system was doing what they were told to do. I imagine that many of the people Sally spoke to wanted to give her the results and understood her increasing fear and anxiety, so they were frustrated with their inability to care for her on a personal level. In addition, insisting on a primary care visit further delays the care and adds an avoidable expense (introducing waste into the system). The patient should have greater choice and empowerment. The excessive paternalism Sally was subjected to makes no sense in today's information-rich world.

What does Sally's experience tell us about who has the power in the health system/patient relationship? It is not the patient. Who controls the patient's medical record? It was not Sally.

Consider the difference in the way we interact with financial institutions. Imagine if you had to ask permission from a bank to view your accounts, get a record of transactions, or move your money to another financial institution. That would be so unacceptable that we would laugh at the very suggestion.

But the opposite is true in healthcare. Instead of owning and controlling her pathology results and reports, Sally had to beg repeatedly even to be told the results. Sally later went to get a second opinion and had to sign a release for *her records* to be sent to her doctor of choice.

The complexity of healthcare should compel us to consider different processes. Processes that are patient-centric and ensure patient care and well-being are always the primary goals.

What if the system was transformed so patients owned their medical records and had to give providers and healthcare systems permission to access them? Think of it like a financial account. That would be transformative, changing the dynamic and placing the power in the hands of the patient as the consumer of healthcare services.

Consumer Focused Processes

Why is it easier to book a seat on a flight from San Francisco to Tokyo than it is to book an x-ray or a doctor's appointment? When we book that flight, we know what seat we will sit in, precisely what the ticket costs, and have an excellent idea of when the plane will depart and when it will arrive. Most importantly, we have great confidence that we will arrive at our destination safely. This is amazing considering we do not know the pilot's name and we may never have flown that airline or been to either airport. As travelers, we have confidence that the system, and the processes that make it function are designed to ensure quality, safety, and reliability even at great distances. The reliability of the airline industry is a testimony to the vision of aviation pioneers and the commitment to continuous quality improvement. Achieving high reliability reflects a commitment to safety, sharing information (including safety data), and transparency that, unfortunately, is inconsistent in our current healthcare system.

High-reliability industries must commit to ensuring processes are as efficient and reproducible as possible. By focusing on process instead of isolated numerical performance targets, leadership acknowledges the myriad of components that must function in a coordinated way to maximize financial realities and value both for the customer and those working within the system. Depending upon its complexity, the system within which processes function must contend with shifting realities, variability, and challenges that the process design and implementation strategies must accommodate.

Those who work on the front lines of the healthcare system know that each patient is unique. The uniqueness of patients is a composite of individual needs, physiologic, genetic, and socio-economic realities. The complexity of patient care is further increased when we consider that each patient enters into the healthcare system largely unpredictably. There is substantial variation in when, how, and where patients seek care, even for the same diagnosis. Therefore, we cannot apply simplistic, reductionist process strategies to patient care and expect to achieve optimal reliability and value. Instead, we must acknowledge and develop processes that allow us to better respond to individual patient needs. The processes we design and implement to provide quality care must function even when confronted with unpredictability within the complex healthcare environment.

Prioritizing the goal of achieving high reliability in delivering healthcare means planning for quality in the long-term and avoiding short-term solutions that cannot accommodate the unexpected. How much effort do we spend "putting out fires" daily? When do those short-term fixes result in sustainable improvement? W. Edwards Deming is credited with saying, "Don't just do things better; find better things to do."[3]

We are arguably at a tipping point in healthcare and need to transform. Continuing to do the same things and expecting different results is not a viable solution to many challenges, from excess cost to waste to inconsistent quality and burnout.

By committing to processes that respect and best understand the individual—providing patient-centric care—we can focus on continuously improving quality and simultaneously providing value by managing cost. In addition, we can better support the ability of healthcare professionals to provide the best care possible, creating reliability even when faced with complexity.

Aspirations of Reliability

I was meeting with the surgery residents one morning to talk about patient safety during their weekly education conference. The discussion was about the relationship between improving communication and patient outcomes. Communication related to patient care, especially a complicated patient, is challenging and involves many different people and teams within and outside the healthcare system. Making communication effective and reliable is a significant challenge from many perspectives, not the least of which is including the patient! Regarding that last point, one resident noted, "We see you give your personal cellphone number to your patients. I would never do that. Don't they call you at all hours?"

I thought about the resident's point and perspective. I had heard that concern before, and I understand it because it is true. I still receive texts and calls from patients I operated on fifteen or twenty years ago!

Why did I give my personal cell number to patients? Because I was not confident in the system's reliability in managing patient communication. Was my approach ideal? Certainly not. A highly reliable system cannot rely upon a single individual to keep it functioning. High reliability, especially in a complex environment, demands consistency and adaptability when situations demand action. To think that one person can manage or should be ultimately responsible for ensuring that tasks are completed within a complicated or complex system is unrealistic and predisposes to error. Unfortunately, these expectations, whether self-imposed or a product of the traditional medical hierarchy and "captain of the ship" mentality, remain common in today's healthcare systems.

High reliability is a concept that has dramatically evolved over the years in different industries, such as the airline, petroleum, and nuclear power industries. Much has been written about the theory behind highly reliable organizations avoiding catastrophic failure. High-reliability philosophy is integral to their day-to-day operations and requires them to consistently provide high-quality products and services to their customers.

When applied to healthcare, the principles remain essentially the same: high reliability requires an organization to be proactive in its safety and quality assurance approach. This means investing in staff training, developing a culture of safety and transparency amongst team members, having detailed documentation systems, and establishing a clear strategy for responding to any incidents or near-misses that occur. High reliability begins with seeing, understanding, and reducing, or at a minimum, managing risk.

Organizations must keep up with changing regulations and technologies related to high reliability. For instance, airlines must stay on top of advances in aircraft design, navigation technology, and changes in FAA rules to ensure their planes comply with all safety standards. Oil companies must invest in high-tech monitoring systems and teams of experts to understand the environmental impact of their operations and minimize risks.

Sharing safety information is essential for high-reliability organizations. In the airline industry, this involves analyzing data from flight recordings and other sources to identify potential risks or issues that need addressing. This process is known as incident reporting, which requires airlines to share safety information with aviation authorities worldwide so incidents can be investigated, and the lessons learned applied across the entire industry.[4]

Remember the Boeing 737 Max aircraft experience? There were two fatal accidents: Lion Air Flight 610 in Jakarta and Ethiopian Airline Flight 302 from Addis Ababa. Despite these accidents occurring in completely different parts of the world, the transparency of data sharing and global commitment to prioritizing passenger safety resulted in the worldwide grounding of all MAX aircraft from March 2019 to November 2020. There is no analogous system in healthcare.

Authors from Johns Hopkins published evidence that medical errors may be the third leading cause of death in the United States.[5]

Potentially preventable medical error is a major public health concern. Despite the frequency of errors, there is no transparency in reporting errors or, more importantly, in sharing ways to reduce risk. The evaluation of medical errors is done within individual centers and, most often, within individual departments. Quality investigations are considered protected and, therefore, not shared with the outside world. Sometimes they are not even shared within the system where the error occurred but kept privately at the department level. While there are standardized approaches, root cause analysis for example, the evidence is that these efforts do not result in sustained improvement. Even if they do lead to improvement, the results, with rare exceptions, are kept closely guarded within the local environment where the quality improvement was done.

To meaningfully improve patient care processes, the investigation of medical error and strategies for improvement must be more consistent and complete and shared like in the airline industry. High reliability will become the norm when healthcare system processes clearly and consistently prioritize patient-centric outcomes.

A Complex Reality

There are aspects of healthcare delivery that are uniquely challenging. Healthcare occurs in a complex environment that is highly interdependent, nonlinear, and never fully knowable. There are often aspects of patient care that are unexpected and unpredictable.

The way patients are cared for within and by the system is a process, and the effectiveness and efficiency are defined as "process flow." Disruptions in process flow significantly impact the reliability and quality of patient care within healthcare systems.[6]

As we will discuss, process flow disruptions cause inefficiency, waste, and increased cost in addition to reducing quality. Resolving process flow disruptions can improve reliability, reduce costs, and improve patient care.

Process flow disruption analysis is a novel approach focusing on system-level strategies to identify and address potential disruptions. This approach involves first acknowledging that the system is complex and, therefore, never completely knowable. Only then can process flow analysis consider the entire system from start to finish to identify areas where disruptions may occur.

As we examine process flow, we must agree on whose perspective the process and system are being viewed from. The goal is to optimize value—the best outcome while managing cost—in providing patient care. It is from the patient's perspective that we must view process flow and identify where the disruptions occur. This may sound obvious, especially for someone who is a patient advocate and who thinks in terms of both individual and population health, but the reality is that this is not always the case.

All too often, for various reasons—including the hierarchical nature of healthcare—the perspective of the process is not from that of the patient. Instead, the perspective may be from the physician (historically the most common), nurse, or administrator—each with their own perspective on improving the healthcare system. The situation becomes even more complicated when these perspectives are biased toward improving their own circumstances. While the opinions of what defines optimal processes from people working with the system may align with the patient's, they often do not.

○ ○ ○

Imagine an eighty-one-year-old who is told he needs knee replacement surgery. The orthopedic surgeon's office schedules the surgery and informs the patient they need "clearance" from other doctors before the surgery date. What exactly does "clearance" mean, and how should the patient get "cleared?" Will one of the physicians, the orthopedic surgeon, the anesthesiologist, or the primary care doctor manage this, or does the patient have to make this happen? Will the hospital take responsibility? What role does the insurance company or government play?

The patient, in this case, has atrial fibrillation and is taking a blood thinner as treatment; he has mild pulmonary fibrosis (scarring of the lungs—the side effect of medication taken years ago), hypertension, and a history of a heart attack four years ago, which left him with kidneys functioning about 50 percent of normal. He regularly sees a primary care doctor and, twice a year, sees a cardiologist, a pulmonologist, and a nephrologist. All these doctors are in different offices and on various electronic medical record systems versions. They may know each other by reputation, but none know each other well. Do the specialists understand the cumulative risk of surgery for this unique patient or the stress a knee replacement surgery and the subsequent follow-up impose on an eighty-one-year-old patient? Also, what socio-economic factors might be in play? Has anyone considered whether the patient has adequate resources for transportation, help at home, or proper nutrition? Does the process ensure all these components are addressed, or will there be disruptions in process flow along the way?

The orthopedic surgeon knows that she needs clearance for surgery, or the anesthesiologist might cancel the case. Finally, what is the motivation for someone recommending surgery? Could the fee-for-service model of reimbursement be an influence? Was physical therapy or other alternatives considered?

Typically, the surgeon's office will contact each specialist and request a letter stating that the patient is cleared for surgery. When a letter is sent, usually by fax, it often states simply, "cleared for surgery."

What exactly does that mean? There is rarely any explanation of risk or specific pre- or post-operative plan. The patient is anxious to have his knee replaced because of pain and limitations of walking resulting from the bad knee and because he has been told: "you need surgery."

If one of the specialists would not "clear" him for surgery, what would the patient and orthopedic surgeon do—likely find another doctor to provide the clearance or try to go ahead without it?

○ ○ ○

In this example, the fragmentation of care is confusing for both the patient and the surgeon. Who is responsible for determining the risk vs. benefit of the surgery? Who takes the time or ownership to discuss risk with the patient? While everyone caring for this patient would acknowledge that he is above average risk, what does that mean, and how does that impact the decision to go ahead with the surgery—which is likely already scheduled? Who documents the discussions with the patient and family? In most cases, no one assumes ultimate responsibility because each team member views the patient through the lens of their specialty. Each specialty has its own process, but none of those are a comprehensive process that follows the patient throughout their healthcare journey. The patient is left to decide whether the proposed surgery is worth the risk involved.

The lack of a process that truly reflects the complexity of the patient care journey from the patient's perspective results in risk that is not fully understood or addressed. The patient must trust that the system process is committed to their safety and that the system will not subject them to unnecessary risk.

The patient journey, the steps from the decision to have surgery to the point of recovery from surgery (which varies from person to person), is an example of process flow. It is certainly not simple! The patient journey through an episode of care is *the process* viewed from a high level. It is where quality, safety, and reliability goals must be placed. Within the patient journey, there are multiple interactions between healthcare system components.

Focusing on limited interactions or sub-processes that are whole components is easier than understanding every aspect of the complex process from the patient's perspective. When portions of the process (patient care journey) are considered in isolation, we falsely assure ourselves that complex processes are easy to understand and control. Isolated, self-limited sub-processes can often be reduced to linear constructs and consequently are assumed to be highly predictable. By focusing on simplified sub-processes, we assume we can "fix" them when they do not work the way we think they should, or at least identify someone to blame when they do not function as expected!

The problem with that approach is that it fails to accept the complexity of the entire process. Efforts to oversimplify can lead to situations where sub-processes are treated as disconnected components of the whole. Furthermore, reductionist approaches change the outcome or key performance indicators (KPI) in ways that might not be aligned with the best patient outcome.

For example, it is common to focus on reducing the length of hospital stay. No one wants to keep a patient in the hospital any longer than necessary. However, from the patient's perspective, hospital length of stay may or may not be related to overall quality. Length of stay is an isolated process measure. To determine the optimal length of stay, we should assess it with respect to quality, safety, and value for the entire patient care process. If the quality of patient-centric care is the primary outcome measure, as it should be, then the length of stay process measure must be assessed with respect to the patient's health at the end of the patient care journey. We must resist the temptation to reduce the patient care process to isolated performance metrics measured for sub-processes.

How, then, should we think about process flow? We have all experienced a sense of accomplishment when a process flows smoothly. At the individual or team level, we might think of optimized process flow as being "in the zone," where disruptions are minimal and human performance is at its peak. We can all think of watching professional athletes having outstanding results when everything seems right—they are in the zone and achieve their greatest success. To be in the zone, extraneous distractions need to be reduced or, ideally, eliminated. If we minimize process flow disruptions, human performance can reach its peak.

At the front lines of healthcare, what the patient perceives as most important is human interaction and performance; providing the best care possible. This is one of the most important elements of the patient experience. Is the professional who is providing care able to understand what the patient is experiencing, what the patient is feeling, and what care the patient needs? From the patient and population health perspectives, process flow should, ideally, be viewed from the patient's perspective. The primary outcome measures of process flow in healthcare must be patient centric. The patient's health, experience, and the value of the services rendered are all important measures of optimal process flow. The impact of process flow on patient care is foundational to meeting the goal of value-based, patient-centric care.

In today's rapidly changing healthcare landscape, process flow disruptions significantly challenge patient safety, reliability, and the ability to deliver value-based care. Process flow disruptions often occur when treatments and protocols fail to respond adequately or consistently to changing patient conditions or circumstances.

In *The Process Manifesto*, we consider the complexity of healthcare systems. We will explore ways to improve the processes designed to optimize patient-centric care. We will consider strategies to help manage complexity. We must become comfortable with understanding that complex systems are dynamic, interconnected, and unpredictable. This requires stepping outside the comfort of many established norms and hierarchies. The call to action is to acknowledge and appreciate complexity and use the Ten Core Principles to optimize process flow.

In doing so, we can *empower healthcare providers to do the right thing for the right patient at the right time.*

CHAPTER 2

MAKING PROCESS FLOW

"A rule of thumb is that a lousy process will consume ten times
as many hours as the work itself requires."

BILL GATES

To improve and increase value from the patient's perspective, each
of us working within the healthcare system must understand the
nuances of process flow and acknowledge that unresolved process
flow disruptions contribute to adverse outcomes and waste. The challenge is to optimize process flow and align the measured output with
patient-centric goals—the best possible health outcome.

At first, it seems simple. Fundamentally, process flow involves a
process's sequential steps. A process flow diagram is a tool used to
illustrate the relationships between major components of a process.
This is especially true for linear processes, which are the easiest to
understand. The classic example is an assembly line.

Creating a linear process flow diagram often begins with a known
result; for example, an automobile. All the components are known,
and the order they are put together is relatively easy to determine.

Working linearly, forward or backward, the process can be diagramed so that each step is described sequentially, and the inputs and outputs of each step are understood. A process flow diagram (PFD) visually represents the steps and decisions needed to perform a process. It provides an overview of all the tasks and relationships involved in a process and helps managers and designers arrange procedures for straightforward outputs. We can assume that in a linear process, the probability of moving from step A to B and further to the end is easy to predict and reproducible. When we create a linear process diagram, we can determine the points where there is the most and where there is the least risk of disruption. Simple probability assumptions can be made.

An example of a linear healthcare process is how a patient moves through a routine clinic visit.

Clinic Visit Process Flow Diagram for Registration Staff

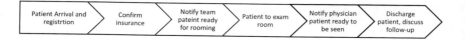

If functioning as a linear system, process flow can be readily described using flowcharts or process diagrams, and they can be adapted for use in a wide variety of applications. Flowcharts are often used to show how different parts of a system interact with each other or how different stages in a project are connected. They can also provide insight into potential problems or areas where improvement is needed. Flowcharts can help teams identify bottlenecks or locations where additional resources may be required, as well as help to visualize complex processes more clearly. By understanding the various elements involved in a process, teams can make better decisions about optimizing their workflow for maximum efficiency.

In a linear process, we can determine the risk of A to B not being complete using predictive analysis or by simply observing the workflow. When process disruptions are observed, we can work backward using failure mode and effects analysis (FMEA) techniques. FMEA is relatively straightforward when something goes wrong in a linear system but becomes increasingly difficult as complexity increases.

A linear process flow is easy to manage because each step's probability of success or failure is knowable. If a problem is encountered, a disruption in the process flow, examining the cause, including root cause analysis, is easy to accomplish.

The desire to increase consistency by reducing variability in healthcare is understandable. Well-intentioned efforts attempting to apply highly predictable and understandable linear constructs to patient care are common. From a management standpoint, reducing care delivery to a linear system is very appealing. What could be better than to understand and think of the process flow of a patient care episode in a structured, linear way—like an assembly line?

The problem with this reductionist approach is that patients do not present or behave like mechanical devices. Individual human beings are not all the same and do not enter the system consistently or repeatably. The unique characteristics and environmental realities that define each of us add an inevitable complexity that does not follow a highly predictable, reproducible, linear construct. This chapter will explore how complexity influences process flow within healthcare systems.

Understanding Process Flow

Process flow is usually divided into two main elements: input and output. Inputs are activities that must occur before any outcome is achieved. In healthcare, these include patient assessment, medical interventions, administrative tasks, etc. Outputs represent the desired result of the process. It is essential to determine the desired output and from whose perspective it is considered a prerequisite for understanding process flow. As the system in which a process occurs becomes increasingly complex, there are inevitably numerous perspectives for what constitutes a desired outcome.

This can be illustrated by considering the various processes involved in a commercial aircraft leaving the departure gate on time. There are many potential process inputs. The passengers must check in, get through security to the gate, and then onto the airplane. The plane must be fueled, cleaned, and catered. The crew needs to be present and qualified for the specific aircraft. The checked luggage needs to be loaded, and the list goes on. Each of these steps has someone in charge, and from their perspective, efficiently and effectively completing the process they and their team are responsible for is the priority; the performance outcome measure they are responsible for, even if they are not necessarily in control of every aspect. If purely linear process models are applied, each sub-process is viewed as largely independent and, at the time of outcome measure, without considering the ultimate outcome measure, which must be a safe flight. Keeping this example in mind, we can consider the challenges when reducing healthcare process flow to a linear construct.

In his book, *The Toyota Way*, Jeffrey K. Liker describes the fundamental management principles that allowed Toyota to achieve its reputation as one of the world's most significant manufacturers.[7] In a linear manufacturing process like building a car, a focus on quality that ensures repetitive processes are as efficient and effective as possible will produce the best results. Process flow is optimized and disruptions are kept at a minimum. When workers notice a process flow disruption impacting quality, they can "stop the line," providing an immediate and dramatic impact to resolve disruptions. Linear processes allow for standards to be applied that are consistent, intentional, and ultimately highly reliable.

Given the success of linear system strategy to improve quality and, simultaneously, efficiency in manufacturing, why not apply the same principles and strategies to healthcare? Using these concepts in patient care is appealing, especially if the goal is reducing costs and increasing efficiency. This strategy is particularly attractive administratively because outcome measures can theoretically be conveniently tied to budgetary priorities. Linear process strategies, Lean and Six Sigma for example, are frequently used by health system departments such as supply chains and pharmacies. Linear process goals include reducing variability and redundancy by increasing standardization. These efforts to impose linear strategies align well with the desire to control costs.

Not unexpectedly, frontline healthcare teams often view these initiatives with skepticism. There are various reasons for resistance to change, but concern about the negative impact of oversimplifying processes on patient care is important. Unfortunately, the promise of limiting variability by imposing tight controls and linear process design has not resulted in widespread healthcare savings. Despite significant and well-intentioned efforts, societal healthcare costs continue to rise, and consistency and reliable outcome measures such as value, safety, and quality in healthcare remain elusive.

Healthcare is Not Linear

Linear system theory is a valuable tool for understanding and analyzing the behavior of many systems. Examples of linear systems include mechanical systems such as conveyor belts or assembly lines; electrical systems such as switches and motors; chemical processes such as fuel burning in a car engine; biological processes such as photosynthesis; and computer networks. Unfortunately, linear systems design does not accurately represent real-world healthcare systems and patient care. Healthcare systems are complex and dynamic, with many intertwined factors that can influence patient outcomes.

Patient safety is a significant concern in healthcare that cannot be fully understood by linear system theory alone. If it could, we would have patient safety outcomes like those in other high reliability organizations like the airline industry. Patient safety relies on multiple interconnected pieces, such as quality measures, patient risk assessment protocols, patient education programs, and patient engagement strategies. Achieving the aspirations of maximizing patient-centric outcomes and patient safety while simultaneously managing (controlling) costs requires more than simply viewing costs and outcomes as always being predictable and reproducible, as linear system theory would suggest. Instead, optimizing healthcare outcomes necessitates a holistic view of patient care that considers patient experience, provider relationships and satisfaction, clinical outcomes, costs, reimbursement, and, most importantly, the complexity of the healthcare system.

Healthcare is complex and reducing it to a linear process will not work. Worse, a reductionist, linear strategy can lead to unintended consequences. A known problem with manipulating isolated aspects of a complex system, such as imposing an overly simplified linear structure onto one system component, is that this can lead to unintended consequences. This is the "butterfly effect."

I have attended many hospital quality meetings where someone proudly informs the group that they have a "Six Sigma Black Belt." These quality experts often point to how they have successfully reduced organizational expenses. Their advice and resultant efforts are typically directed at reducing specific cost center expenses, for example, pharmaceuticals, devices, or labor. Discussions tend to emphasize reducing variability. These initiatives usually identify the least expensive alternative that presumably provides equivalent results when implemented.[8]

Fair enough, no organization wants to spend more money than necessary. Underlying these cost-saving initiatives is, ideally, a belief that there is a moral and ethical imperative to ensure optimal patient-centric outcomes. *First do no harm.* However, the challenge is that the ultimate decision-makers are, from a practical perspective, often not involved in providing direct patient care. Their performance is measured not by specific patient outcomes, but instead by KPIs tied to budget expectations.

The interface between cost-center management and clinical care providers is variable and not standardized. Typically, the people responsible for reducing expenses communicate with physician and nursing leadership, who agree that costs need to be controlled. Manager and leader job security and promotion within a system is often tied most strongly to financial performance. Due in part to the small margins within important components of our healthcare system (for example, many hospitals), the easiest way to achieve positive short-term financial goals is to cut expenses. Since, at least in the United States, our healthcare expenses have increased to levels that many consider unsustainable, who could disagree that the cost of care needs to be reduced?

To reduce expenses for the hospital, the decision support team will provide healthcare team members evidence that less expensive alternatives are "just as good." Whether the data available is comprehensive, applicable to all patients equally, and without bias is often suspect. Product substitutions rarely undergo a rigorous process, including testing or even an evaluation period. It is not unusual that product decisions result from contracting, including through global purchasing agreements. Few healthcare organizations have the resources to assess such decisions' consequences continuously and seldom consider the butterfly effect.

I remember one example. I performed laparoscopic, minimally invasive pancreas resections when the technique was first established. At the time, the standard was to do these operations through a large incision in the abdomen. The laparoscopic technique eliminates the large incision and the resultant pain. Pancreas surgery is always challenging. Anatomically, there are large blood vessels around and within the pancreas, including the artery to the spleen and the splenic vein. A criticism of the laparoscopic technique was the concern that if there was bleeding from a large artery or vein, the patient could be at risk of serious complications, even death. In the traditional open technique, the surgeon places a clamp on the blood vessels, then divides (cuts) them and oversews the ends of the artery and vein with vascular suture. Over the years, this technique has been proven to be safe and effective. Because it was new, safety data for laparoscopic pancreas surgery was not comprehensive nor widely accepted.

When the surgery is done laparoscopically, the surgeon divides the main artery and vein using a vascular stapling device placed into the abdomen through a small port. Using a camera placed through a separate port, the surgeon, looking at a TV screen, squeezes the stapler handle. This simultaneously sets rows of metal staples and cuts through the blood vessels with a knife blade that the surgeon cannot directly see. The surgeon releases the handle of the stapler, and if everything is as expected, there is no bleeding, and the artery and vein are divided. Success!

More than one company makes laparoscopic staplers, and there are differences between them in the design, the way they work, and the number of staples put into the tissue. The operating room team (me, residents, nurses, and scrub techs) had used the same stapler for two or three years. We were experienced using it and were satisfied with the results, both in the OR from the perspective of ease of use and reliability and, most importantly, from the excellent patient results. No patient had ever experienced significant bleeding nor had to return to the operating room post-operatively.

The challenge for the surgeon, and by extension, the patient, is that the surgeon rarely has any meaningful say in which manufacturer's stapler the hospital or health system purchases. In addition, the staplers may be changed suddenly to a different manufacturer if the supply chain business unit signs a new contract for a better deal—typically because the cost per device is less. When changes are made, with rare exceptions, there is no opportunity or time for training outside the clinical space, and certainly never as a team.

In my case, I had a patient scheduled for a laparoscopic distal pancreas resection on Monday. The Friday before, in the late afternoon, an email was sent by the hospital's chief executive office and leadership team to all surgeons stating that the hospital was changing stapler manufacturers. The entire stock of staplers was to be removed over the weekend, and the new brand put into use Monday. Even as the chair of surgery, I was never asked my opinion. I and the other surgeons were just expected to go along with the decision. The hospital leadership's email assured us that the supply chain committee had studied the literature and made a wise choice. The email did not state that the primary reason for the change was to save money, although we all suspected this was the case. Interestingly, while we all understand the need to manage costs, I do not know of any example where surgical supply cost savings translated into a lower surgery price for the patient. The final reassurance in the email was that the new manufacturer's representatives would be in the operating rooms on Monday and Tuesday to provide support.

My patient was brought to the operating room on Monday. The

operating team completed the surgical checklist and we introduced ourselves. Interestingly, the checklist did include a question about equipment, but none of us considered the substitute stapler significant. Notably, there are no standards for informing the patient about equipment substitutions or changes. Patients are rarely, if ever, informed. That may reflect the paternalistic nature of medicine. It is assumed that the patient does not have the knowledge (or the right?) to make informed decisions regarding what medications, equipment, or supplies will be used. The patient certainly should have confidence and trust that the medical team will ensure that the most appropriate items will be available and used during care and that the team knows how to use those items. In fairness, that is a foundational tenant of high reliability.

The surgery began as usual. The case proceeded routinely to the point where the stapler was needed to divide the artery and vein. The manufacturer rep was in the operating room as promised. She was engaged and enthusiastic, but I had never met her, nor had any other team member. She showed the scrub nurse how to put the staple and knife blade cartridge into the stapler handpiece. At this point, although focused on a problematic aspect of the surgery, I became concerned. From the conversation, it was clear that the scrub tech was uncomfortable with how the stapler worked. Why had we not been trained to assemble or use the stapler before being in the OR with a patient? Unfortunately, this happens all too often. It is assumed that a new device is similar to what was used before, so no time or resources are provided for meaningful additional training. In the hospital, especially in the OR, training is done "on the job" while a patient is being operated upon. The patient is never told this.

○ ○ ○

Consider if the airline industry had the same approach. Imagine being fortunate enough to be flying business class from Chicago to Paris. You are in your seat, sipping a glass of champagne as you wait to depart on the vacation of a lifetime. The cockpit door opens, and you see the pilot and a maintenance person. They are talking about a new GPS device just purchased because it was less expensive than the equipment they had used for daily transatlantic flights for many years. The maintenance person is installing the new GPS into the cockpit, removing the existing one. As you watch this scene, the pilot states, "I have never used this GPS before."

The maintenance person replies, "Neither have I, but we received an email saying they reviewed the literature, and it works just as well."

If I heard this conversation, I would be concerned, wondering why no flight crew member had been thoroughly trained on the equipment. If this did occur, I would probably get off the plane!

Of course, we know that the airline industry and regulatory bodies like the Federal Aviation Administration would never allow this. The pilot and crew would all need to be trained, most likely in a simulated environment, on the new GPS before it was installed in the aircraft and used. In healthcare, we substitute devices, medication, and sometimes protocols with little notice and usually without additional training.

○ ○ ○

In the case of the pancreas resection, I inserted the new stapler into the abdomen. The rep advised me on how to use it, and I placed it around the artery and vein and squeezed the handle. When I released the stapler, the end of the artery looked like a sprinkler — spurting blood in multiple streams with each heartbeat. Fortunately, I was able to remove the stapler device rapidly and had a backup vascular clip applier opened and ready to use. The nurse gave me the clip applier, and I stopped the staple line bleeding with only a couple of ounces of the blood being lost. The patient did well and had an uneventful recovery.

There is no standardized reporting of events like this in healthcare. In reality, they are rarely, if ever, documented. No data was collected and assessed for this event (a near miss) or similar ones that occur daily. A high-reliability organization would classify our experience with the stapler as a "near miss." Yes, my patient did well. Unfortunately, we, and more importantly, the healthcare system, did nothing to learn from it. Nothing was done to prevent it from occurring again in the future. If it did happen again, would the outcome be the same, or might the patient have a serious complication?

The stapler did not perform as expected in this case, disrupting the flow of the operation. We accept events like this as "a known risk." We are conditioned to ignore flow disruptions if they do not result in a severe adverse consequence. This myopic view fails to acknowledge the potential for implications within a complex system that we do not understand. Our experience and perspective are limited and do not usually contribute to improved outcomes at a higher system level. The consequences of our limited, myopic view are likely not understood or known.

Flow Disruptions

Events that disrupt process flow come in many forms. The substitution of the laparoscopic stapler is one example. There is usually enough resilience in the system to avoid catastrophic failure or sentinel events, instead resulting in a "near miss" or an error that does not result in demonstrable harm to a patient. Unfortunately, we have come to accept a degree of disruption as a relatively routine aspect of the day-to-day work in healthcare. There exist people within our healthcare system who openly accept some baseline level of disruptions to flow and the error that results as inseparable from routine healthcare operations. We hear comments that justify mistakes, such as "a known complication, recognized and managed appropriately." End of discussion. If someone pushes back and questions whether things might have been done differently, they may be viewed as "disruptive" themselves!

Process flow disruptions cause a break in the primary process or task. They can severely impact the efficiency and effectiveness of an organization's operations. Flow disruptions exacerbate the fragmentation of patient care, affecting the local environment or system level, or both. They can be caused by various factors, from external sources to internal issues.[9]

Process flow disruption analysis is an approach to direct quality initiatives emphasizing system-level strategy. It involves identifying and analyzing the factors that cause disruptions and then developing strategies for mitigating them. Flow disruption categories can include many factors ranging from small to large, such as procedure type, patient group, or even population. The analysis is designed to understand each factor's impact on the process. A descriptive flow disruption model is used to understand better how the disruptions affect complex processes and operations. This model can be used to identify potential areas for improvement and develop strategies for mitigating risk.

Process flow disruptions are best analyzed and understood from the perspective of the ultimate outcomes measure; patient-centric care for example. It is essential to recognize and address process flow disruptions to ensure efficient and effective operations within an organization. The challenge for those responsible is to avoid the inclination to reduce the global process into overly simplified subunits with misaligned performance and outcome measures.

The Patient Journey

Suppose we follow an individual patient care process (patient journey) from start to finish. Process flow can be viewed from multiple perspectives within the patient journey, whether brief or extended. Each perspective may differ significantly when determining what is necessary to achieve an acceptable outcome. Team members may not even agree on an acceptable outcome, further complicating matters.

From the patient's perspective, the process involves all steps, from diagnosis through treatment and follow-up. Every step is subject to flow disruptions, and each can directly impact patient safety and outcome. Process flow disruptions are interruptions that prevent efficient and effective care delivery and may contribute to waste and error, two important contributors to avoidable costs. To reduce process flow disruptions, healthcare organizations must design and implement processes for care delivery that focus on ensuring the quality and reliability of care. Optimal processes can simultaneously manage and even reduce healthcare costs.

By addressing process flow issues, healthcare organizations can ensure the best possible experience for their patients and improve patient safety, outcomes, and value.

Process flow disruptions undeniably have financial implications for healthcare organizations. The costs associated with process flow disruptions can be significant. They include extended wait times, additional labor costs incurred due to rework and delays, increased administrative and legal expenses for resolving claims issues caused by process flow errors, and many more. Furthermore, process flow disruptions can lead to missed opportunities for revenue, such as when a patient needs help accessing needed services due to process errors or even a lack of processes designed to accommodate unpredictable patient needs.

Communication

Strategies to resolve process flow disruptions cannot begin without effective communication. Healthcare organizations have recognized that they can improve patient safety and value-based care by fostering timely and accurate communication. What can be improved upon is consistently relating efforts to enhance communication to optimizing patient-centric process flow.

Communication across and within a complex system's components is essential for efficient and effective processes. Communication occurs in many forms, including verbal, written, and electronic. Effective communication must be relevant to all involved, regardless of its form. Communication should reinforce goals and objectives that are understood and agreed to by all involved. Distracting and unnecessary or irrelevant communication can be a process flow disruptor. Keeping every team member focused on the high-level outcome goals (i.e., patient-centric outcomes) helps ensure that communication is clear, relevant, collaborative, accurate, and timely.

Improving communication to minimize flow disruptions requires education and training. It cannot be assumed that everyone is a communication expert. Effective communication, especially in a high-reliability organization, is a learned skill that must be refined and practiced. Optimal communication strategies change over time, for example when new regulations and new technologies are introduced.

Much of the effort to improve communication within healthcare systems has been focused on interactions that are considered disruptive. While it is true that poor communication can be disruptive, including to process flow, the effort to improve communication has tended to be punitive. Rather than focusing only on people considered disruptive due to a history of poor communication, teams function better when communication skills are improved for all. This requires consistent education, training (including simulation), and importantly constructive feedback.

Evaluating communication and the factors affecting communication, such as misaligned priorities or distractions, should be included in investigating adverse events. Highly reliable organizations must ensure that communication is effective.

Given the complexity of the patient healthcare journey, the process inevitably involves many different system components. The diversity of people and teams involved in patient care challenges communication. These challenges are exacerbated when priorities are not aligned because the information communicated may be important from one person's or a single team's perspective, but of little utility for another.

Inconsistent and poor communication can be confusing from the patient's perspective when they expect everyone "to be on the same page." This often leads to reduced patient satisfaction and unnecessary anxiety. One strategy to overcome this is to understand what communication the patient and members of the health system team require to optimize process flow. Effective communication can help to coordinate care and make the patient journey through the system more reliable. Improving communication is an effective way to reduce the negative impact of separate departments or independent system components. At its best, communication facilitates the ability of teams to work effectively together to optimize process flow.

Teamwork

In a process-oriented complex environment, teams of teams are becoming increasingly common. They provide a structure for completing tasks and projects and help ensure everyone works together towards the same goal. A team of teams in a process-oriented environment work by breaking down tasks into smaller, more manageable chunks and assigning them to different team members. This way, each team member can focus on their specific area of expertise while still contributing to the overall project. The team of teams structure allows for adaptability when faced with unexpected, unpredictable situations. This approach decentralizes decision-making, helping to create a more patient-centered healthcare system. Decentralization can be challenging for people more comfortable with a hierarchical structure. Hierarchy is a traditional element of our health system, making decentralization a disruptive challenge to the status quo.

However, as we will discuss, managing processes in a complex environment requires decentralized approaches designed to empower professionals on the frontlines to perform at the highest level possible. Empowering the front-line care teams minimizes process flow disruptions, and optimal outcomes are achieved.

To be successful, a team of teams must have several key features in place. First and foremost, healthcare teams must have clear, patient-focused, measurable objectives. This is true even if the team is not directly involved in patient care at the front line. The team members should be familiar with the specific goals they are working towards and understand how each person's role contributes to the larger mission. Functions should be clearly defined to clarify who is responsible for what tasks or decisions. Communication between team members must be effective and frequent to ensure everyone is on the same page.

Secondly, teams of teams need patient-focused, trusted, collaborative, and flexible leadership. Leaders need to balance patient needs and business goals, develop a shared decision-making process, and adjust when needed to meet patient needs. Putting the patient's needs first is necessary to avoid prioritizing efforts to performance metrics limited to a single operational unit or department. Additionally, leaders should foster an environment where everyone feels comfortable contributing ideas or concerns without fear of repercussions. An effective team of teams structure ensures that the expertise of each team member is incorporated into the function of the whole. Each team's contribution to the process must be understood from the other teams's and the patient's perspectives. A clear and consistent focus on quality outcomes coupled with effective communication and sharing of information is critical to accomplish this.

The success of process-oriented teams is dependent upon communication. Team members must be able to communicate effectively with each other to ensure that everyone is working towards the same goal. Communication can come in many forms, such as meetings, emails, phone calls, or even text messages. Team members need to stay up to date on any changes or updates so that they can adjust their plans accordingly.

Another critical aspect of process-oriented teams is collaboration. Each team member should feel comfortable sharing ideas and opinions to develop creative solutions and task-completion strategies. Trust among team members is essential for any successful team dynamic. Process-oriented teams need to have clear goals and objectives that everyone can agree upon and strive towards achieving together. This will help keep everyone motivated and focused on completing their tasks on time while ensuring that all team members are accountable for their contributions.

Teams of teams need processes in place that promote patient safety, quality, and value. This includes ensuring patient data is secure and accessible to all stakeholders involved in the patient care process flow. Processes that guarantee patient involvement throughout the care process strengthen and support the decentralized model. The patient must feel that the team of teams is working for and with them.

Continuous Team Improvement

Process flow improvement teams are essential to the success of optimizing patient care in a complex system. In a practical, real-world example, we created a surgical services quality committee that consisted of teams of teams. The structure of the quality committee followed International Organization for Standards (ISO) 9001 standards.[10] Every member received ongoing education to ensure all knew about ISO 9001 strategies and the outcome measures being used. The ultimate measure of success for every process flow improvement project was a patient-centric outcome. The committee consistently identified process flow disruptions and inefficiency by utilizing a team-based approach. Strategies were developed to improve processes. The committee included a broad constituency that extended well beyond the surgery departments and operating rooms. Membership included diverse departments such as environmental services, pharmacy, primary care, geriatric care, and hospitalists.

To maximize the diversity of opinion and experience, we used a unique approach to place experts in one patient care area into teams assigned to process improvement where they were not normally involved. For example, an orthopedic surgeon was placed on a team focused on robotic general surgery, and a general surgeon was placed on a team focused on spine surgery. This effectively reinforced one of the core principles of the team of teams approach, bringing expertise into new or unusual situations where their knowledge and experience can provide a different perspective, reducing bias. The team of teams approach encouraged members to view process flow in new ways, exploring new innovative solutions.

The quality committee confirmed that the team of teams approach could help optimize processes, reduce costs, and improve patient outcomes. Leadership provided clear objectives and goals and the resources needed to achieve them. The team had access to data and analytics to help them identify improvement areas.

When the team identified potential improvement areas, a process flow plan was developed and tailored to the organization's needs. Monitoring progress on an ongoing basis is essential. The Plan-Do-Check-Act model is perfectly suited to continuous monitoring and quality improvement. The decentralized team of teams model encourages continuous assessment by those on the frontlines of patient care. This facilitates rapid intervention if the outcome improvement goals are not being achieved or if the process improvement strategy has unintended consequences. Regular meetings or other forms of effective communication with all team members can help ensure issues are addressed quickly and efficiently.

It is important to ensure that patient and stakeholder feedback is actively sought and used to provide insight into how well the process flow improvements work. Feedback to the teams is important, celebrating successes achieved by process flow improvement teams and providing a positive incentive to improve process flow continuously. The effort to improve process flow, especially in a complex environment, is always dynamic and inseparable from the philosophy of continuous quality improvement.

CHAPTER 3

MAKING SENSE OF SYSTEMS

"A bad system will beat a good person every time."
W. EDWARDS DEMING,
"FOUR DAY SEMINAR WITH DR. W. EDWARDS DEMING"

No one would argue against the statement that healthcare delivery occurs within a system. We use the term "healthcare system" in our daily conversations. Despite the everyday use of the term, there is no uniform or consistent definition of a healthcare system. Our perspectives of what makes up "the system" depend on our focus. From a public health perspective, the system contains populations that can be relatively small and well-defined or extremely large, even global in extent. From the individual patient perspective, the healthcare system refers to the components of care delivery that impact them during an episode of care or, more broadly, over time. That likely includes, at a minimum, insurance, physicians, and access to medications and hospitals. The healthcare provider most often considers the healthcare system as the resources they need to deliver the best care to their patients. One might also add the myriad of things physicians and other caregivers need to deal with, such as insurance networks and pre-approval, hospital system-imposed restrictions, government regulations like HIPPA, electronic medical records, etc.

No matter the size and scope of the healthcare system, the processes that occur or should happen within the system matter most when we focus on patient-centric outcomes, including quality, safety, and value. To optimize the process of delivering care and establish the highest reliability, we must understand what type of system we are working in and how the system is functioning. We can describe a system as one of three types: simple, complicated, or complex.

Comparing Types of Systems

Simple or Linear	Complicated	Complex
Elements are known and interactions are controllable	Multiple elements function together in coordinated way (the system is sum of components)	Relationships are nonlinear Small change in one element can result in large change in another (butterfly effect)
Known knowns	Known unknowns (disassembly / retrospective analysis can identify unknowns)	Unknown Unknowns (never completely knowable)
Inputs results in predictable outputs (deterministic)	Historic function of system predicts future outcomes	New patterns of system function occur spontaneously (emergence)

Simple or Linear	Complicated	Complex
The process is consistent, few changes over time	Expertise necessary to understand cause and effect and to optimizing function	Expertise is essential but does not guarantee predictable outcomes Discretion is needed due to dynamic situations that change over time
Related processes do not affect each other (independence)	Subsystems interact in known ways	Subsystems are interrelated and interactions are not fully knowable
No direct feedback loops	Feedback loops exist, can be managed, and help identify solutions allowing control	Feedback within system variable Positive increases effect of change, negative reduces effect of change

Linear Systems

When it comes to health system process improvement and process management, linear process or system theory is the one most often employed. A linear system follows the principles of superposition and homogeneity. This means that when input signals are applied to the system, the output will be a linear combination of the inputs. The two main characteristics of linear systems are homogeneity and time invariance. Homogeneity states that if you multiply all inputs by a constant, the output will be multiplied by that same constant. Time invariance says that the result will remain unchanged if you apply the same input at different times.

If healthcare were a linear system process, a patient would always enter at one point in the process, and the process, if strictly followed, would produce a predictable, desired result. Administratively, this construct is appealing because it should be easy to identify waste and sources of error. This is a reductionist view of the healthcare world. Anyone who cares for patients knows that no two patients are identical or seek care under the same circumstances; there is too much variability, even if the eventual treatment plan is the same. Patient variability is due to multiple etiologies, including overall health, genetics, and socio-economic and environmental realities.

Even with intra-patient variability, components of a patient's healthcare journey can, in theory, be reduced to linear sub-processes. These tend to be simple, routine, and reproducible processes such as registration, insurance verification, and confirming that the correct procedure is being done. In linear processes, checklists are effective tools to help ensure all process components are considered and available. From the perspective of the front-line healthcare provider, and the patient for that matter, patients are all unique human beings, and therefore, patient care is rarely, if ever, linear and predictable.

Linear process flow, because it is predictable and consistent over time, can be analyzed to identify errors, bottlenecks, and sources of waste so that they can be rectified and improved. In healthcare facilities and systems, LEAN and Six Sigma are popular approaches to process improvement. At the risk of oversimplifying, LEAN emphasizes eliminating activities that do not add value directly to a patient's care process and Six Sigma focuses on optimizing processes through statistical data analysis.

LEAN and Six Sigma both originated in the manufacturing sector. LEAN, often called Lean Management, is a systematic approach to process optimization developed in the twentieth century to reduce waste and improve productivity and quality. The Toyota Production

System (TPS) originated in Japan in the 1940s and 1950s and is often considered the birthplace of many LEAN principles. Toyota's key figures, including Taiichi Ohno and Shigeo Shingo, developed it. LEAN strategies are particularly effective when industries face resource constraints and economic challenges. Toyota leaders were able to use LEAN to innovate and find ways to do more with less, implementing techniques such as just-in-time production, kanban, and continuous improvement. In the 1980s and 1990s, the principles and practices of TPS were introduced to Western manufacturing industries. This is when the term "LEAN" began to gain prominence as it was translated and adapted for Western contexts.

Six Sigma was initially developed at Motorola in the 1980s. The credit for its creation is often attributed to Bill Smith, an engineer at Motorola. He aimed to improve manufacturing processes by reducing defects and variations in products. The name "Six Sigma" refers to a statistical term representing a level of quality that allows only 3.4 defects per million opportunities, in other words, a highly stringent quality standard. The Six Sigma philosophy spread to General Electric in the 1990s, gaining significant prominence when Jack Welch, the CEO, adopted it as a core part of the corporate culture, emphasizing data-driven decision-making and process improvement.

Over time, LEAN principles expanded beyond manufacturing and found applications in various sectors, including healthcare. Virginia Mason Medical Center in Seattle, Washington, and Toyota Memorial Hospital in Toyota City, Japan, were early adopters who played a crucial role in popularizing LEAN in healthcare. Although there are some differences between LEAN and Six Sigma, they share fundamental philosophies and the implementation of both is similar, especially at the frontlines of healthcare.

When applied to healthcare to improve process flow, LEAN and Six Sigma's significant emphasis is identifying and eliminating perceived waste, including unnecessary steps, redundancies, and delays in healthcare processes. Ideally, this leads to streamlined work-flows and improved efficiency and encourages healthcare providers to focus on delivering value to patients by reducing errors, improving the quality of care, and enhancing the overall patient experience.

LEAN/Six Sigma proponents promote the development of standardized work processes, procedures, and protocols designed to reduce variability in care delivery and make it easier to maintain quality standards. When adequately supported, the implementation of standards includes continuous improvement or Kaizen. Healthcare organizations use this to foster a culture of ongoing evaluation and adjustment to ensure that processes are continually refined.

Continuous quality improvement is an essential, foundational element for the success of both LEAN and Six Sigma. Quality improvement teams can use various strategies, including DMAIC (Define, Measure, Analyze, Improve, Control), and PDCA (Plan, Do, Check, Act). These strategies provide a systematic framework for improving processes by defining objectives, measuring performance, analyzing data, implementing improvements, and establishing controls to sustain gains.

To succeed, continuous quality improvement must be adequately supported in terms of time, money, and personnel. While cost reduction is a significant benefit of LEAN, focusing solely on cost reduction may inadvertently lead to sacrificing the quality of care. Support of quality improvement and process optimization includes data analytics and expertise. Expertise includes salary support for physicians and nursing staff. The cost of this support can be a challenge for organizations and, unfortunately, is often seen as non-essential, therefore being a frequent victim of budget cuts. Quality experts, especially senior physicians, are often seen as unnecessary costs that do not generate revenue, especially in a fee-for-service environment.

In addition to justifying the cost of quality experts, especially at the senior level, LEAN and Six Sigma have other limitations when used to improve processes in healthcare. If we agree that healthcare is inherently complex, with numerous variables and unpredictable patient conditions. Overly standardized approaches may not always accommodate the variability and complexity of medical care. Trying to reduce every patient to a uniform standard analogous to a linear manufacturing process is not realistic nor reflective of reality.

Another challenge is that organizations may become overly focused on achieving specific metrics and targets, potentially leading to a fixation on numerical goals rather than genuine process improvement. This can create a "metrics-driven" culture that neglects other important aspects of operations. There is no practical way to enforce rigid standardized processes and individualized, patient-centric care simultaneously.

Optimized processes clearly need evidence to support them (i.e., evidence-based care) while also being flexible enough to respond to individual patient needs. Overly committing to unvarying, manufacturing-style processes fails when managing in a complex environment.

For those responsible for leading and managing healthcare delivery, an appeal of linear process theory is that it is relatively simple to explain, describe, and understand. Linear systems allow for the relatively straightforward implementation of policies and procedures and, if believed necessary, corrective actions. Linear processes are easy to diagram on paper and assign accountability or responsibility to various process steps. Linear thinking assumes high predictability and, by extension, high reliability if the people interfacing with the system adhere to the system as designed. This construct includes the belief that the people working within the linear system must conform to the rules (policies and procedures) deployed to control the system as it is defined.

Administratively, using linear system thinking is appealing because of the ability of management to identify deviations from the predicted linear process expectations and ascribe responsibility when the system does not work as designed. Unfortunately, the assumptions inherent in linear system thinking can be used to assign blame (which, to some, is a synonym for accountability) when the linear process does not function as expected.

Applying linear system theory to healthcare process design can help leadership to manage or control costs and, at the same time, meet patient safety and quality expectations. Managing these potentially conflicting outcome goals within healthcare is difficult. Therefore, applying linear system theory seems like a perfect strategy. If linear system management has demonstrated success when applied to highly predictable and uniform processes such as building cars, why not use the same approach when caring for patients? I have listened to many presentations that focus on isolated aspects of the patient journey that do often follow linear processes, such as registration or room turnover time between procedures. Unfortunately, when committed to achieving linear outcome consistency, the strategy tends to fall short of expectations.

○ ○ ○

The operating room committee is a real-world example of the problems associated with expecting linear system theory to work within the complex healthcare environment. As a young surgeon two years out of training, I was excited about my appointment to the university hospital operating room committee. I thought, "what an honor!" At my first committee meeting, the entire hour consisted of a discussion about why the first case-on-time start metric did not reach the 80 percent that the consultants had proposed as an industry norm. All of our twenty-three operating rooms were expected to start at the same time, 7:30 a.m. There is no uniform definition for OR start time, but most often, it is when the patient is brought into the operating room.

This discussion lasted more than the hour allotted to the committee meeting. I realized that most of those sitting around the table believed someone else was to blame. Only 60 percent of our first cases of the day were on time. The surgeons blamed anesthesia for not being prepared; the anesthesiologists blamed the inconsistency of the pre-operative information; the operating room managers blamed the surgeons for always being late. This circular firing squad discussion dismayed me since there were no winners.

Furthermore, I thought to myself, how practical is it to think that twenty-three operating rooms can all start at precisely the same time in the morning when there were so many variables? The surgeries performed in the various rooms had very different personnel and equipment needs. In addition, the risk potential was different, for example, between a straightforward cholecystectomy and a living donor kidney transplant. To expect both to follow a highly consistent start time did not make sense. Applying linear process metrics to a complicated or complex situation did not seem realistic. If the operating teams' performance was measured primarily by metrics like first case on-time start, what happens to the patient quality and safety goals? Do those become secondary to time-based linear performance expectations?

To me, the expectation that twenty-three operating rooms could start simultaneously was impractical, if not impossible. As an analogy, consider if the discussion was about an airport instead of an OR. What would happen if the airport management set the expectation that the first departure from each gate must be at precisely 7:30 a.m.? That would certainly create gridlock and result in delays, if not chaos. So why should we think that the operating room first case on-time start was a valid metric for measuring healthcare team performance?

What relevance did the on-time start outcome measure have to patient safety or quality?

As I walked out of that first long and contentious meeting and reflected on how disturbed I was by what I had heard, the chair of anesthesia, a senior faculty member nearing retirement, put his arm around my shoulder. "What did you think?" he asked.

I replied, "Well, I must admit it was not what I expected. I thought we would discuss something related to improving patient care."

He smiled and said, "Doug, the OR Committee is like a soap opera. The same things are discussed year after year without any solution or resolution. You can be on the committee this year, then off for five years. When you return, the topics and discussion will be the same. You will have missed nothing!"

Now that I have been a member of many OR committees in several hospitals during the past twenty-five years, I can say, disappointedly, that he was 100 percent correct.

Limitations of the Linear Approach

Despite continued enthusiasm, linear process or system theory has significant limitations when applied to healthcare systems and patient care processes. Healthcare services are more complicated than traditional manufacturing processes due to the inherent variability among individual patients and unpredictable influences such as patient socio-economic factors. Individual patient-level variability makes process design, management, and improvement far more complex than an assembly line. Additionally, linear process or system theory assumes that processes are static when healthcare services often require rapid changes in the process flow that cannot be effectively managed via traditional process improvement approaches.

Furthermore, linear process or system theory relies heavily on metrics that are integral to the process to measure success. For example, a success measure in a linear assembly line process could be the percentage of time a particular step is completed correctly (like the first case on-time start). Since the steps in a linear process are deterministic and predictable, a measured failure rate can be ascribed to a specific step in the process and corrected. This is quite different from many patient-centric outcome measures used in healthcare. Many patient care outcome measures are more subjective and difficult to quantify, especially from the patient's perspective; being pain-free or having a good quality of life, for example. Those measures tend to be highly individualized.

Ultimately, while linear process or system theory has some applications in healthcare systems, its limitations must be acknowledged. Linear process or system theory can be a valuable tool for process improvement and process management in healthcare organizations for standardizable patient experiences like clinic check-in or validation of insurance. These are examples of highly repetitive and routine tasks. However, it is essential to recognize the limitations of linear, reductionist process design due to the complexity and variability of patient care and the difficulty of quantifying process success. Organizations can make more informed decisions about improving their services by understanding the advantages and drawbacks of using linear process or system theory when managing healthcare processes.

Complicated Systems

A complicated system has many components, each interacting with other components to achieve a desired outcome. A complicated system's essential characteristic is its many interdependent parts and processes that must be coordinated to function correctly. The components tend to act in patterned ways and normally behave predictably. A car engine is comprised of hundreds of components that must work together to run correctly. Similarly, a computer network consists of many interconnected computers and devices that must communicate with each other for the network to operate efficiently.

Complicated systems can be managed in ways that make safety a priority. For example, commercial air travel today is remarkably safe and reliable. The system supporting air travel is complicated, but the steps necessary to safely get a plane from the departure gate to the destination are predictable and manageable. That is not to say it is easy. The United States has over 45,000 flights and over 2.9 million airline passengers daily.[11] The tremendous work to keep the system safe, given the volume, the myriad of components, and variables such as weather, must be coordinated at many levels.

In a complicated system like commercial aviation, a completely centralized model of control would never work because of the inability to respond effectively to local environmental realities. Those responsible for leading and managing system components must collaborate and work to eliminate individual operating unit silos through communication and transparent data sharing. The common principle that underlies the operational strategies employed is a commitment to safety at all levels. Remarkably, the last fatal commercial fight in the U.S. was in 2009. Contrast this with the National Institute of Health's estimate that there are up to 98,000 avoidable inpatient deaths annually![12]

One reason for the success of commercial aviation is an acknowledgment that the system is inherently complicated (as opposed to linear), and that the system is managed with a consistent focus on safety as *the comprehensive measure of success*. The strategy for managing a complicated system contrasts with prioritizing individual component outcome metrics, as can happen when reduced to a linear system model. When safety is prioritized above the outcome measures ascribed to the individual sub-processes of a system model, including in complicated and complex systems, the outcome can be remarkably dependable.

Successful management of a complicated system includes adaptability. This means the system can adjust itself in response to changes in environment or user input. For example, the recognition of wind shear preventing a safe landing can trigger a delay in departure hours before. In this example, the safety of the passengers and crew is more important than an on-time departure (which would be an isolated quality measure—easy to obtain, but not directly related, and perhaps contrary to a safe outcome). Another example is that an automated factory may be able to adjust its production process based on changes in customer demand or new technology being introduced into the market. Similarly, an online store may be able to adjust its pricing structure based on changes in customer preferences, demand, or economic conditions.

Finally, another key characteristic of a complicated system is its resilience. This means it can continue functioning even when some components fail or are removed from the system. For example, if one part fails, then other components may be able to take over its role until it can be repaired or replaced. A complicated system must have adaptability and resilience to function correctly and achieve desired outcomes.

An example in healthcare would be a patient having a CT scan of the abdomen ordered due to persistent abdominal pain. The patient arrives as scheduled for the test, and the only CT scanner available is under repair. The person at the registration desk knows that the department also has an MRI machine that could provide the same information. In a linear system model, the test would be canceled for that day, and the patient would be told to go home and reschedule. The priority in this example is to complete the task as defined. In contrast, if the process was designed using complex system strategies, the priority would be to ensure that patient care was optimized, and a diagnosis made. Applying the concepts of adaptability and resilience, the person at the registration desk would be empowered to see if the alternative of an MRI scan was possible in a time frame that made sense for the patient.

Complex Systems

"... whatever we do affects everything and everyone else, if even in the tiniest way. Why, when a housefly flaps his wings, a breeze goes round the world."
Norton Juster, *The Phantom Tollbooth*

Complex systems are a fascinating phenomenon studied in many fields, from biology to physics to engineering. A complex system comprises many elements that interact dynamically, for example, by exchanging energy or information. These interactions can lead to behaviors and outcomes that are not easily predicted or understood. Some relationships and resulting outcomes may be unknowable in a complex system, even when using advanced analytics or AI.

The first characteristic of a complex system is its nonlinearity. This means the system's behavior is only sometimes predictable. It can be and often is highly unpredictable and even chaotic. Unpredictability makes it difficult to anticipate the outcome of any given interaction between elements within the system. Another characteristic is emergence. Emergence refers to the ability of a system to produce new behaviors or outcomes from interactions with other elements within the system. For example, when two simple aspects of a system interact in a complex way, they can produce a result not expected from either factor alone.

If interactions between elements within a complex system are not considered when designing a process flow, optimizing outcomes is difficult, if not impossible. This is not to imply that things can be controlled as in a linear system, but rather that leadership must acknowledge that to achieve optimal outcomes, the processes in a complex system must be able to respond to uncertainty. Rigid assumptions and strict control are not effective when managing a complex system.

Instead of rigid policies and procedures, processes within complex systems need to be resilient. Resilience allows systems to respond to the unexpected, especially adversity, when there is no ability to control an outcome. Professional expertise, competency, purpose, and flexibility contribute to resilience when dealing with complexity. Resilience can take the form of spontaneous problem solving, and if focused on a clearly defined goal, can effectively maintain process flow when faced with disruptions.

A third characteristic is a spontaneous order. Spontaneous order occurs when a group of elements spontaneously organize themselves into patterns without any external influence or control. This type of organization often leads to unexpected results. It can be used to explain phenomena such as flocking birds or ant colonies working together towards a common goal without any central coordination.

A fourth characteristic is adaptation. Adaptation refers to the ability of a complex system to change its behavior in response to changes in its environment or inputs from elements within the system. This allows for more efficient use of resources and greater resilience against external shocks such as natural disasters or economic downturns.

Unpredictable and unexpected events happen in healthcare. They can be challenging but finding a way to understand a complex patient presentation, adapt, and alter care to meet the individual patient's needs is one of our profession's most rewarding and fulfilling aspects. Years ago, I was told the story of a patient who happened to be a nurse. She had donated a kidney to her daughter. The surgery was routine, as was the postoperative course, and she was discharged to home within a day. Her first follow-up clinic visit was unremarkable. She was doing well, and all her incisions were healing as expected. About two weeks later, she returned to the clinic with wound infection in the incision made to remove the kidney for transplantation. Over the next month, the transplant team tried every routine to treat the infection and get the wound to heal. Nothing seemed to work, and the patient was becoming increasingly frustrated. The transplant team was similarly frustrated because the patient was not getting better.

Finally, they arranged for home nursing to do daily dressing changes. After the first visit, the home nurse called the transplant coordinator. She said that there were more than twenty animals in the house, including cats, dogs, and ferrets, and that they were sleeping in the bed with the patient, and she suspected licking the incision. Now the team understood the reason for the persistent infection. A new treatment plan was made, the infection was cured, and the incision healed.

Response to Risk

This level of complexity is not unusual. The patient's interactions with their environment and other factors, such as socio-economic and cultural realities, often challenge our healthcare system to adapt and accommodate. This is especially true when trying to understand and manage risks before they result in an adverse outcome. How would the different system theories manage process flow to respond to changing and unpredictable risk?

A linear response (often the most likely approach) would be to create a policy stating that patients cannot be around animals after surgery. This policy would be duly recorded and filed away, along with hundreds of others, to be dusted off when the next such complication occurred or when the transplant program regulators showed up to review all policies. It would likely be attached to an email that all team members had received. The responsible manager would be secure in knowing that they had "checked the box" regarding appropriate follow-up and a process was in place. Everyone is happy, but has anything changed?

The reality is that the policy by itself is unlikely to be followed consistently or effectively, reducing the risk of infection. When the next patient with animals at home returned to the clinic with an infection, the blame would be placed on the patient or some unfortunate team member who forgot to ask and tell the patient about the policy. This is the problem with linear process thinking applied in a complex environment. The process outcome metric is a new policy instead of patient outcome. In applying linear process theory, nothing has meaningfully changed, and the outcome metric is not patient-centric, instead being the process itself.

If complicated system theory were applied, an evaluation of dressings would likely be undertaken. There are more expensive alternatives that prevent animal saliva from getting on the incision and would likely reduce the risk of infection. The question is how to use this more expensive item best. The easiest approach is to have every surgeon use the new dressing for every patient. This would be a costly approach. Considering that the overall infection rate for this type of incision is one or two per one hundred operations for all patients, and that the circumstances experienced by this unique patient is much less, using a more expensive surgical dressing for all patients does not make economic sense. Even if chosen as the solution, it would not be long before the supply chain experts prohibited or severely restricted the use of the more expensive dressing. The supply chain department might stop purchasing it altogether.

Applying complex system theory, the healthcare team would assess whether there was an increased risk of infection *before* the surgery. You could ask the patient if they had animals, how many, and if they slept in the bed. The patient may or may not answer honestly, and even if they were honest, it is unlikely that they would remove the animals from their house around the time of surgery. A transformative approach would incorporate a data-driven analytic solution that assessed and included factors such as medical history, home environment, and socioeconomic status. We have all experienced searching for something on the internet and subsequently received ads related to our search or targeted advertisements for things in our life, like pet supplies. By extension, including that level of information could help the care team identify risk and better manage it prospectively.

Complex system theory argues for providing for a selection of resources, such as the more expensive incision dressing, so the frontline healthcare provider can select the most appropriate choice based on knowledge, experience, and—most importantly—data. If the provider, at the time of care delivery, had actionable information (data) demonstrating increased risk and the resources available to mitigate that risk, the process flow would be improved, and the probability of a better patient outcome would increase.

The fifth characteristic of complex systems is feedback loops. Feedback loops occur when an output from one element becomes an input of another component within the same system, creating a cycle that can amplify certain behaviors or outcomes.

The sixth characteristic is self-organization. Self-organization occurs when individual elements within a system interact to form patterns without external direction or control from outside forces such as humans or computers. This type of organization often leads to unexpected results that may be positive or negative. Finally, complexity itself is also an essential characteristic of complex systems. This means that these systems are composed of many different elements interacting with each other in various ways, which makes them difficult to predict and understand fully. Complexity can increase the probability of unexpected results. At the same time, complexity affords great potential for producing insights into the world around us if managed appropriately.

Managing Process

Processes are essential to providing patient care and treatment promptly and effectively. Implementing LEAN process management and linear process flow has been widely advocated for healthcare organizations to improve quality, reduce cost, and to achieve the best patient outcomes. The primary goal of LEAN process management is to focus on eliminating waste by streamlining organizational processes for improved efficiency. One can see the influence of the supply-side of healthcare. The theory is that if you can control the use of products and supplies, then variation is reduced, and costs can be controlled. While this might be philosophically appealing, healthcare costs have certainly not decreased, quite the opposite! The complexity of our healthcare system, which includes competing, misaligned interests, reduces the effectiveness of linear process management strategies.

Linear process flow uses structured steps to organize tasks into a step-by-step process with predetermined outcomes. These concepts are often used when creating healthcare processes because they offer standardization across departments and easily trackable process flows. However, some researchers argue that implementing overly standardized processes may increase disparities in care instead of reducing them.

One explanation is that a standardized approach cannot accommodate patient variability resulting from complex factors, including genetic, physiologic, behavioral, and socioeconomic, which in combination make up a patient's healthcare need and response to care. If only one standardized care pathway is available, some patients will inevitably be left out or not experience optimal outcomes.

Adhocracy

On May 25, 1961, before a joint session of Congress, President Kennedy stated that the United States "should commit itself to achieving the goal, before this decade is out, of landing a man on the Moon and returning him safely to the Earth."

The goal was achieved on July 20, 1969, when Apollo 11 landed on the Moon's surface.[13]

The goal for NASA was clear: land a man on the moon. Professionals and experts were assembled by administrators who themselves were not experts in the field; the administrators were not, after all, rocket scientists! The administrators knew their responsibilities, and the complexity of the task, so an adhocracy was formed instead of establishing a bureaucratic, centralized control model. The belief was that if you put a group of experts (the rocket scientists) together and gave them a clearly defined goal, they could effectively use resources to find solutions to situations or problems that emerge.

The administrators realized that the complexity of getting a man on the moon was daunting. There was a need to adapt, innovate, and develop solutions organically, quickly, and efficiently. Experimentation was necessary. In addition, the administrator recognized that they had to avoid turf wars between competing branches of the military that functioned as silos.

Bureaucracy and adhocracy can be considered opposites in many ways. A bureaucracy tends toward centralized control with rules and systems that cover everything. An adhocracy (from the Greek "ad hoc," meaning for the purpose, and "cracy," meaning to govern) is inherently more flexible and decentralized.

Let us consider aspects of adhocracy as strategies to improve process design in the complex world of healthcare. For example, establishing a clearly defined goal like landing on the moon. If we agree that patient-centric outcomes are that goal, then the professionals working within the system know the priority. Our healthcare systems are plagued by competing priorities that strongly influence system-level organization, structure, and process. This is one of the reasons thought leaders argue for a single-payer system—to remove at least some of the competing priorities and conflicting incentives that exist.

By virtue of being decentralized, adhocracy tends to facilitate employee engagement and communication within and between teams. Professionals are empowered to self-organize into teams of teams to achieve the primary goal (i.e., patient-centric care). Examples of this are seen in some specialized centers, such as those managing cancer and transplant patients. Improved engagement of professionals at the point of work can ameliorate burnout, frustration, and dissatisfaction with an overly rigid, unforgiving work environment.

Administratively, there are challenges with adhocracy, some of which are philosophical. Processes may become more difficult to control because they adapt to the unexpected in an adhocracy rather than conforming to a centralized norm. It becomes more difficult to hold individuals accountable for failure. On the other hand, the professional team can identify poor performance more rapidly and intercede at the operational level when there is a recognized problem. Incompetence is more difficult to hide in an adhocracy where the frontline is empowered more than in a large, centralized bureaucracy.

There are additional costs involved in adhocracy. For example, increased education and training are needed to optimize professional competency and performance. Increased reliance on technology, including data analytics, is also necessary to ensure processes function as designed. Continuous quality improvement based on measurable agreed-upon outcomes is essential.

When healthcare delivery is overly standardized and controlled centrally, the individual receiving care may not receive the best treatment for their unique needs. Standardized processes and systems are designed to provide a one-size-fits-all approach, which can lead to suboptimal outcomes for patients with specific health conditions or needs. Linear systems and linear process management cannot account for individual patients' differences, as they do not allow for customization of care. Instead, the healthcare team must consider each patient's unique circumstances to ensure they receive the best care. Providers must balance standardization and personalization to deliver higher value in health care. Standardization can help streamline processes and reduce costs in linear processes, while complexity requires flexibility to ensure that each patient receives tailored care based on their needs.

If optimizing patient-centric outcomes is agreed upon as the overriding priority, then the leadership must establish processes that do not restrict but instead empower those on the frontline of patient care. When empowered by leadership, healthcare providers are more likely to deliver high-quality care while also being able to consider cost. Empowerment requires actionable information combined with education, training, and experience. By leveraging technology and finding ways to customize care while maintaining efficiency, healthcare organizations can provide value by ensuring optimal patient outcomes and simultaneously optimizing the use of resources to manage expenses.

Complex process flow is the most flexible type of process management system, as it involves interactions that cannot be easily defined or categorized into distinct steps. Instead, this system relies on self-organizing models that allow dynamic adjustments based on changing conditions and unpredictability. Complex system process design can accommodate changes in conditions since it allows for process deviation when necessary. Living with and thriving in complexity has many advantages. However, tracking and managing processes can be challenging due to the resistance to conform to standardization.

Ultimately, process flow decisions should be based on a healthcare organization's specific environment and goals. Linear process flows may offer an effective solution in organizations with simple process requirements, while more complex process management systems may be necessary for organizations dealing with highly variable conditions. By understanding the differences between linear, complicated, and complex process flow, healthcare providers can ensure they are making informed decisions when selecting process management strategies.

Applying Complex System Management Theory

Healthcare systems are complex. Many autonomously functioning components work in various degrees of coordination to provide patient care. Complex system management theory can be applied to healthcare systems to improve patient care by creating more efficient and effective processes. This theory can be used to identify how knowledge is captured and used clinically at the point of care delivery.

The components of the system that are needed to provide optimal care vary, including for different patients having the same diagnosis. The effective management of a complex system requires that interactions between system components are optimized and occur at the right time to be most effective. When linear models attempt to control each component of a complex system, the ability to coordinate and align resources with individual patient need is difficult. Feedback loops and strategies that foster synergies (like creating a team of teams) should be encouraged when managing complexity. Leadership must resist isolating processes into silos.

To effectively manage complexity, leadership must encourage communication and transparency between operating units, healthcare providers, and patients. The processes developed within a complex system must incorporate a greater understanding of the relationships between healthcare system components. Forming teams that include members representative of system diversity is an effective strategy for managing complexity. This reduces the disconnectedness associated with silos and instead encourages collaboration and teamwork. Applying complex system management theory within healthcare systems can help create an environment where all stakeholders can access the same information and work together more effectively. By understanding how different components interact, healthcare providers can better identify areas where improvements can be made continuously.

Complex management theory incorporates the principles of continuous quality improvement for optimizing patient care processes. The same processes create an environment where the patient care team is empowered to be adaptable and use the resources available most effectively. Processes created using complex management theory include feedback loops that ensure actionable information is readily available in real-time to the professionals who need it to perform at the highest level. By relinquishing top-down control and eliminating overly restrictive processes, leadership supports an environment that increases collaboration and communication between team members.

Complex system management theory can reduce errors in patient care by providing a better understanding of how different components interact with each other. To facilitate this, outcome metrics and KPIs must be aligned. The ultimate quality metric must be agreed to, acknowledged, and shared by all key system stakeholders. Assuming we agree that the ultimate quality metric will be patient-centric outcomes, then through processes that strengthen relationships within the system, healthcare providers can identify potential problems before they become serious issues and take steps to prevent them from occurring in the first place. This could include implementing processes for double-checking medical records or introducing new technologies (telemedicine, remote patient monitoring, automated patient engagement, etc.) that allow for better communication between those working within the health system and between the care team and patients.

In 2011, Gökçe Sargut and Rita Gunther McGrath published an article in the *Harvard Business Review* titled "Learning to Live with Complexity."[14] This article examines how organizations can strategically cope with the demands of a complex environment. The authors argue that complexity should be embraced and managed, not feared or avoided. They suggest that organizations use a combination of structure, processes, and culture to create an environment conducive to dealing with complexity. The article outlines several strategies for managing complexity. These include creating a shared understanding of the organization's goals and objectives, establishing clear roles and responsibilities, developing effective communication channels, and leveraging technology to streamline processes.

Additionally, the authors emphasize the importance of fostering an organizational culture that encourages learning and experimentation. By embracing these strategies, organizations can better manage complexity while achieving their goals.

Applying Complex System Theory Key Points

- A patient's healthcare journey is rarely, if ever, a straight path.
- Complexity has always existed but now touches everyday life in ways unknown a generation ago.
- Reducing variability by assuming every process is linear and highly predictable has limited applicability if patient-centric outcomes are the priority.
- Process flow must acknowledge that individual patients have different personal circumstances, behaviors, and realities that change over time.
- Complexity in healthcare may exceed our capacity to understand it fully.
- Unexpected results of interactions within a complex system are to be expected (the butterfly effect).
- Actionable data and analytics are essential tools to help manage complexity effectively.
- Complex systems have the challenge that patients having the same starting condition may have very different outcomes.
- Complexity is best managed by establishing teams of teams and empowering those on the frontlines to use their education, training, and experience most effectively.
- Optimal processes should (will!) deliver the proper care to the right patient and the right time.

CHAPTER 4

CHECKLISTS AND PROCESS FLOW

"Always do what is right. It will gratify half of mankind
and astound the other."

MARK TWAIN, *NOTE TO YOUNG PEOPLE'S SOCIETY*, 1901

Experts in system theory have recognized the effectiveness of checklists in improving the process flow in all types of systems. Checklists become increasingly important as complexity increases. They are a powerful tool for streamlining processes and ensuring every step is noticed and remembered. They provide a clear list of tasks, reminders, and other information to improve patient outcomes by reducing errors and improving accuracy. By carefully considering each step in a process, healthcare team members can ensure that all appropriate measures have been completed before moving forward with patient care.

Checklists are an essential tool for ensuring consistent patient care and improving safety. They have been shown to help reduce medical errors, improve patient outcomes, and enhance communication among care providers. In his book *The Checklist Manifesto*, Atul Gawande makes the case that checklists can be especially effective in complex clinical settings due to their ability to capture the nuances of unique patient needs and circumstances.[15] The 2009 publication by the Safe Surgery Saves Lives Study Group and co-authors demonstrated that when checklist protocols are correctly implemented, they enable better coordination between healthcare teams, ensure critical steps in the process are not missed, provide structure for communication around diagnosis and treatment decisions, and offer important reminders about context-specific issues that may otherwise be overlooked during a procedure or treatment episode.[16] Checklists also serve as a tool for self-assessment, allowing healthcare teams to identify potential risks and adverse events before they occur.

When applied to linear processes, well-designed checklists are easy to use and create. They can be quickly adapted to any healthcare setting. When used correctly, checklists provide a simple yet effective way of streamlining processes, reducing errors, and improving patient outcomes. By clearly outlining the steps for patient care and related procedures, checklists help ensure that the correct procedure is being done. By using a well-designed checklist, clinicians can be confident that the resources needed to provide high-quality care are available, including the right people, skills, equipment, and supplies. Because checklists are designed to be verbal, communication between team members is improved. Safety, reliability, and effectiveness improve if the checklist appropriately supports the process.[17]

While checklists are a powerful tool that can improve process flow, even in a complex environment, they can only be truly effective if appropriately designed and used consistently and correctly. Checklist design should focus on ensuring optimal patient outcomes.

Checklists can help improve communication between healthcare providers. By providing a common language for discussing patient care, checklists can facilitate collaboration between departments and ensure everyone is on the same page regarding patient care. Checklists should ensure the adequacy and alignment of resources and expertise. If implemented before a process or procedure being initiated, checklists can reduce the incidence of process flow disruptions. To be effective, this requires that each team member is empowered to voice concerns and that the entire team agrees upon the outcome metric with the highest priority. The highest priority should be centered on the patient. Unfortunately, this is not always the case. Conflicting priorities can interfere with checklist use and efficacy. Team members might feel pressured to begin a procedure without adequately completing all the checklist steps or simply ignoring key components. For example, they may feel they have inadequate time to complete the checklist. Team members are often distracted by other tasks they must complete, and those may compete for time that should be devoted to the safety checklist. Team members may even be out of the room gathering supplies that they did not have time to do during a short room turnover between patients.

Unexpected events or emergencies can also interfere with checklist completion. When faced with an emergency, using a checklist designed specifically for emergencies would make sense. Still, most often there is only one checklist; a standard designed for routine, elective cases.

Despite the advantages of checklists in the complex healthcare environment, and research demonstrating effectiveness, there remains room for improvement in the consistency with which they are used. Many healthcare team members remain skeptical, even cynical, about the benefits of checklists. It has been stated that when asked, most physicians say they would want a checklist used if they were the patient, yet many still do not consistently use checklists or take them seriously when the tables are turned. The question is, why? Cognitive biases such as the illusion of invulnerability and normalization of deviance can hinder checklist use. These psychological phenomena lead healthcare workers to overestimate their capabilities and underestimate the importance of checklist compliance. Another factor to consider is how checklists are created and used. If they are not perceived as helping to improve process flow or reduce error, checklists may not be taken seriously.

The surgical checklist is often called a "universal protocol" within healthcare organizations. Does it make sense that every surgery, from an eight-minute cataract procedure to an eight-hour liver transplant, would have the same checklist to ensure the critical elements are in place for an optimal outcome? Would an airline use the same checklist for every aircraft, from a small regional jet to a Boeing 787?

How do checklists get created in most hospitals? Usually, a group is assembled to create a checklist that meets regulatory guidelines and established norms. At best, this group will be members of the team who will ultimately use the checklist. Training regarding checklist design and implementation is important but may not occur.

The group will create a checklist with the necessary elements to meet approval by various stakeholders and possibly regulatory agencies. The length and detail of a checklist can vary. The checklists are rarely, if ever, tested in a simulated environment; instead, once approved, they are implemented "universally." The most common metric used to verify success is the percentage of time the checklist is documented as being completed. Whether the checklist functions to improve patient outcomes is not routinely assessed.

Another reason for checklists not being used correctly or taken seriously is that the outcome measure has shifted from improvements in patient care (as in the original research) to documenting the completion of the checklist. Currently, the most common success metric related to the operating room checklist is the percentage of time the checklist is documented as being completed. If the goal is to complete the checklist instead of achieving the best patient outcome, then the value of the checklist is diminished.

If the team's focus becomes the documentation of checklist completion, then we can understand why team members might rush through the process, skipping steps. The outcome measure of any process, including a checklist, is critical to its acceptance and appropriate use. External performance pressures, such as operating room throughput, reduce the likelihood of checklists being used as designed. A checklist should help the team identify any increased risk of process flow disruption, such as missing equipment or supplies. When taken seriously, a checklist empowers the team to pause or stop the process until the deficiency is resolved.

Checklists should be a tool that is adaptable to unique situations that arise. This is consistent with the complex system management theory. Rigid standardization can impose limitations and may decrease the relevance of a checklist to a given situation.

Well-designed checklists help teams to identify potential hazards or problems before they occur, allowing them to take corrective action as needed. Checklists can also be used to evaluate performance after each patient care process. By reviewing the checklist, healthcare team members can identify areas where improvements may be needed and adjust accordingly. This helps ensure all team members perform at their best and minimize potential risk. Checklists provide an effective way to stay organized, understand the resources available, and prepare for possible problems, ensuring safety is always the top priority.

Situational Awareness

Situational awareness is necessary if teams are going to function cohesively and at peak performance. Being aware is inseparable from process flow optimization. Situational awareness is recognizing and understanding what is happening around you. To be aware of your situation is to be informed, alert, and knowledgeable about what might change as time goes on.

Situational awareness includes the ability to comprehend the local environment, the process you are involved in at the time, and the larger system in which you are working. Having situational awareness means that you can anticipate future needs and respond more effectively to changes or disruptions in the flow of a process. For a healthcare team, situational awareness is, ideally, a shared experience where each team member contributes and supports others in ways that optimize the final outcome.

Situational awareness is within all of us to a certain degree, but ongoing education and training have been shown to improve individual and team performance. Unfortunately, in healthcare, we have not embraced regular training, for example, in a simulation center, to reinforce team performance and situational awareness. This type of training is expensive and requires a culture committed to team-oriented performance. Incorporating and emphasizing situation awareness as a checklist design and use component can be a powerful way to optimize process flow, especially in complex situations.

Checklists can be useful in improving situational awareness in several ways. They provide a structured method of gathering information and assessing the local environment. Checklists can help move decision-making from reactive to proactive, emphasizing preventative process improvement. Improving situational awareness increases team performance in managing complexity, including recognizing risk and potential error.[18]

When using a checklist, it is important to understand that resources, the environment, and the situation are not rigid or fixed in time or space. This might seem obvious, especially if we agree that healthcare is complex. The critical interplay between checklists and situational awareness illustrates a challenge in managing complexity. To be effective, checklists must empower teams at the point of care delivery to be able to adapt and respond. A "one size fits all" approach that attempts to apply rigid standardization cannot be expected to work within a variable and complex environment.

When using a checklist, the team must be confident that they will not be penalized for acting to mitigate risk and ensure safety as a priority. There must be alignment between the checklist, the team actions, and the outcome measures used to determine performance. A checklist can be most effective if the ultimate outcome measure is patient centric.

Information

The usefulness and efficacy of checklists is strengthened when everyone involved has access to the information they need to perform their work effectively. Actionable information is important, especially for those on the frontlines of providing care. Information is different from data, which needs interpretation and analysis. One objective of a checklist is to remind the team to ensure they have the correct information to proceed safely. For example, ensuring that the right patient is getting the correct procedure. The proliferation of electronic medical records has increased the ability to access data. Still, more is needed to provide the most up-to-date and complete *information* to the healthcare team at the point of care delivery. Analytic methods such as machine learning and AI are starting to be used in ways that can support the healthcare team in understanding how the patient care process can be optimized at the time. By accessing relevant information, individuals can make better decisions and take appropriate action when required, making checklists even more effective.

Limitations

Checklists are a great tool to help us remember and organize tasks, but they have limitations. First, healthcare checklists are rarely tested before being implemented. They are often designed using reverse engineering. Creating a hospital checklist often begins with the desired outcome, for example, ensuring the correct procedure is being done for the patient, then the steps necessary, or thought to be necessary, to achieve the desired outcome are added to the checklist. Regulatory guidelines further influence checklist design. A method to ensure the checklist produces the desired result should be part of the process for approval. A simulation environment would be ideal for testing, but this is seldom used.

To ensure they are effective, checklists must be validated and continuously improved to remain current. Checklists should be re-evaluated after every incident or near miss, revising them as necessary.[19]

As mentioned, checklists may be too rigid and not allow adaptability in certain situations. If a task requires creative problem-solving or involves complex decision-making, there may be better approaches than a standardized checklist.

Checklists can be time-consuming to create and maintain, and they require careful thought and planning to ensure that all tasks are accounted for and everything is noticed. Checklist design and review require expertise that may not be available in every organization. Guidelines and additional resources can help organizations optimize checklist performance.

Checklists can become too long or complex, making them difficult to use effectively. If a checklist is overly detailed and too long, it can lead to confusion or frustration when attempting to complete the tasks on the list. The opposite can also be true. A checklist might be too short and leave out important process steps. These are reasons that checklists should be tested and monitored over time to ensure they function as intended and produce the desired outcome.

Checklists can only achieve desired results if used correctly and consistently. Ensuring everyone involved in a process understands how the checklist should be used and follows it accordingly is vital. Team organization and culture must be supportive and aligned with checklist use. This can be a challenge! Collecting and sharing outcome information can reinforce the commitment to use checklists. Checklists can be an invaluable tool when used correctly and consistently, but they have limitations that must be considered.

CHAPTER 5

SYSTEMS AND SILOS

"All things appear and disappear because of the concurrence of causes and conditions. Nothing ever exists entirely alone; everything is in relation to everything else."

THE BUDDHA

How can systems theory be applied to healthcare to improve patient outcomes and increase value in healthcare systems? Systems theory is a way of looking at the world, including the one we work in, emphasizing the interconnectedness of all parts rather than just looking at individual components. When applied in healthcare systems, we must consider the interactions between different system parts, including patients, providers, administrators, insurance, policymakers, and other stakeholders. We must seek to understand the relationship of component parts that might not be inherently obvious, and which have unknown and uncertain influence on the system. Only by understanding, or at least considering, how different components interact is it possible to identify areas where changes can be made to improve patient outcomes and increase value in healthcare systems.

Appreciating how different parts of the system interact makes it possible to improve process flow within the system. If we accept that healthcare systems are inherently complex, the challenge for us is that the interactions between system components are not highly ordered or consistently predictable. Complex systems are not fully knowable. This concept is uncomfortable for most of us and contrasts with strategies emphasizing control and reducing variability as the solution to fixing healthcare.

Suppose we try to apply the reductionist approach and force linear system management principles to control complexity. In that case, we are left in a position where things often seem to function differently than expected. We develop workarounds to accomplish tasks that fixed routines do not effectively accommodate. An example is the "curbside" consult that physicians rely on to share information necessary to care for patients because the system does not adequately support them in other ways. In a worst-case scenario, we constantly struggle to "put out fires." Unfortunately, this happens daily in healthcare—anyone working in a hospital can recount many examples.

Suppose we embrace complex system theory and strategies that work with—instead of opposed to—complexity. By doing so, we can improve reliability and empower the frontline caregiver to be most effective at ensuring that process flow is smooth and produces the best result.

Complex system management is hampered by organizational structures that break down the system into separate units. Admittedly, it is much easier to manage areas of a healthcare system individually. In doing so expertise is concentrated. It is easier to define the work being done when individual components or departments are viewed in isolation from the whole. Specific performance metrics can be defined and readily applied to individual departments. Budgets are also simplified.

While there are valid reasons to reduce complexity by isolating individual components, creating silos, this approach does not reflect the patient's healthcare journey or experience. Patient outcomes are the sum of the interactions of all the silos they pass through during any specific episode of care. In addition, the total cost of care is not defined by any one system component in isolation, as every patient knows all too well.

The siloed nature of healthcare is a frequent source of complaints from both healthcare providers and patients, and rightfully so.[20] Let us explore how complex system theory can reduce the barriers created by silos.

Impact of Silos

Healthcare systems are becoming larger. They are undeniably complex and challenging to manage. One challenge is that the components of the system are most often managed separately and largely function as independent units. Within healthcare, we use the term "silos" to describe different operational units independently operating. Silos exist in various forms throughout our healthcare system, whether our perspective is from the population/societal level or the individual hospital or clinic. Historically operational units within hospitals and medical centers were developed based on professional training and expertise and were therefore defined primarily by specialty or service. Clinical departments are prominent examples. Other departments, such as nursing, environmental services, pharmacy, and purchasing (supply chain) tend to function independently. Individual hospitals can be seen as silos even when part of a larger system.

A consequence of department and other silos is that decisions tend to concern internal unit perspectives and performance measures. The day-to-day workings of the independent management model affect frontline caregivers who have little input or ability to change the structure. Silos frequently are a source of frustration when trying to align resources with patient care needs.

Creating siloed operational units makes sense if one is trying to reduce complexity to manageable components. In this model, departments and operational units function under asynchronous key performance indicators (KPI) that can be cross-purpose and therefore misaligned. This leads to problems when processes focused on patient-centric quality are proposed. For example, a quality initiative benefiting one operational unit (silo) may increase the budget in another silo. Even if the overall or total cost of care is reduced, a silo with an adversely impacted budget will likely argue strongly against the quality initiative and find justification for not supporting it.

One example is a project developed to reduce patient readmission after spine surgery. A multidisciplinary team reviewed the factors associated with unplanned readmission following spine surgery. A process that included innovative risk assessment, patient engagement, and remote monitoring technology was developed. The proposal convincingly illustrated improved patient-centric quality measures, including decreased readmission. As expected, there was an upfront cost for the new technology, but the return on investment (ROI) analysis demonstrated that the total cost of care would be reduced. Further, readmission after surgery is a publicly reported patient safety indicator, and improving this is aligned with system goals.

There were two significant hurdles to overcome. First, which silo would assume the cost of the new technology? This was problematic and contentious. The quality department did not have an independent budget, and with respect to technology was beholden to information technology (IT). IT had invested heavily and was committed to the electronic medical record (EMR) software. The IT leadership was adamant that the EMR could somehow do the things proposed by the quality team. The quality team evaluated the EMR but found it did not meet their needs relative to this project. The IT silo successfully protested the proposed innovation as hurting their budget, preventing the project from progressing.

The second hurdle to overcome was the silo related to individual hospital budgets. Under the existing fee-for-service model, readmission after spine surgery was reimbursed and contributed a significant revenue stream to hospitals with a high volume of spine surgery. If readmissions were reduced as predicted, some hospitals would experience a loss of revenue. Certainly, there is an ethical and moral reason to improve patient care by improving quality. Still, the negative impact on the hospital budgets meant that new investment was not feasible. The quality team was told that the initiative to reduce readmissions was admirable but that no operational unit could afford the cost.

There is one more piece to the puzzle of this quality initiative. Assuming it was funded, who would be the ultimate beneficiaries? The patient is the primary beneficiary because of the improved quality of care. The patient experience and outcome were the primary goals of the quality team that developed the project.

Remember that in addition to improved quality, the financial analysis predicted the total cost of care would be reduced. The beneficiary of the reduced total cost is whoever pays for the care; in most cases that is an insurance company (whether private or government). Recommendations regarding optimizing the financial healthcare system model are beyond the scope of this book, but as this case study illustrates, aligning the payment model with patient-centric care is critically important.

This quality improvement proposal illustrates the impact of silos on global initiatives. From a practical perspective, the flow of money is where silos intersect. Suppose each silo functions independently and budget considerations have management priorities that do not consistently align with patient safety, outcomes, and value of care. In that case, innovations such as reducing readmission may be difficult to implement.

From the perspective of delivering patient care, budget silos limit collaboration between departments. Because each department has a budget, there is an incentive to increase revenue and reduce expenses without fully realizing the impact of decisions on other units, or more broadly, on patient outcomes. This can lead to inefficient use of resources that may not be aligned with the patient journey, resulting in higher costs overall.

Patient-centric care suffers when departments cannot collaborate effectively because they compete for revenue. The patient journey passes through different departments. If each functions independently as a silo, care becomes fragmented and providing patients with the optimal, most cost-effective, and efficient resources is difficult.

Without an accurate picture of how resources are used, and money is spent across the patient's journey through the system, it is difficult to identify areas where resources could be better utilized. Correcting this requires a consistent and accurate understanding of the patient experience. Strategies to reduce the negative impacts of silos at the system level include information sharing and transparency to identify opportunities for efficiency improvements that result in cost savings.

Complex system management strategy should avoid creating an environment where departments compete. Competition between departments can lead to increased tension and a lack of trust between team members, impeding collaboration and communication. Competing departments can lose sight of the entire patient journey and the goal of optimizing patient care. Managing complexity requires that siloed operational units work together towards common goals.

A Shared Vision

The mission of a healthcare system should be to provide effective and efficient patient care that delivers value by optimizing outcomes and, at the same time, managing cost. Complexity imposes many challenges for teams working toward these goals. By its very nature, a complex system imposes significant communication and coordination challenges. Unintended consequences frequently arise, which go unresolved if one functional unit does not see the impact of decisions on other departments. Managing complexity requires departments and operational units to share a vision and culture that unites them in achieving the highest level of performance. A common point of reference is required. The communication of vision, purpose, and information must reinforce the priority outcome measures. When a common goal is established and agreed upon, trust between departments and the people working within them increases, allowing people to begin to make sense of complexity.

By breaking down silos, organizations can create an environment where employees are more likely to collaborate and share ideas. This can lead to improved efficiency, better communication, and increased productivity. One way to break down silos is by encouraging open communication between departments. This could include regular meetings or brainstorming sessions where employees from different departments come together to discuss their projects and ideas.

Being diverse and inclusive of as many stakeholders as possible strengthens the teams, especially multidisciplinary teams. How do you identify relevant stakeholders? Try using the patient's perspective.

Everyone who interacts with a patient during their episode of care is part of the process. When establishing a system-wide surgical quality group, we included many departments not normally considered relevant to surgical quality. The standard members would include anesthesia, various surgery department leaders, operating room nurses, and the operating room manager. These are certainly important team members, but consider surgery from the patient's perspective. For the patient, the surgical experience includes many others, such as primary care, registration, environmental services, hospitalists, social workers, physical therapists, billing, and so on. Managing complexity requires moving beyond our immediate sphere of influence and acknowledging that the process from the patient's perspective involves many interdependent components. To understand how complexity affects a process we are involved in, we must view it not from our individual perspective but rather from the perspective of the whole, including the ultimate outcome measure. Whenever a patient is concerned, the outcome goal must be patient centric.

To reduce the negative influence of silos, leaders should foster a culture of collaboration where everyone feels comfortable sharing thoughts and opinions. The surgical quality committee leveraged collaborative teamwork to identify and resolve process flow disruptions. The group's work resulted in feedback loops that fostered innovation and empowered people to solve problems as they encountered them. Because of the inclusiveness of diverse stakeholders, many of whom previously did not feel engaged, word of successful process improvement spread rapidly. The engagement was further enhanced through a collaborative that included monthly webinars sharing information and best practices. These were done live and recorded to maximize the number of people who listened to them. In less than six months, the number of people engaged grew from less than a hundred to over 1,200 across multiple hospitals.

Education and Training

The surgical quality initiative's success demonstrates the ability of teams, empowered by ongoing education and training, to improve process flow in a complex environment. Improving processes within a complex system requires that leadership support people on the front lines to optimize human performance. Using adult learning theory, education, and training is powerful and effective if relevant. Relevance to a shared objective is important if people are to commit time and effort. Goal setting and ownership of outcomes are important if adult learning is to be effective in supporting process improvement. The relationship between adult learning and complex system management starts to become clear when we consider the need to have people to perform consistently at a high level; to make full use of their professional training and experience.

When initiatives designed to improve patient outcomes incorporate adult learning theory, the key components of process improvement are reinforced. Providing education and training, and incorporating it into the system's culture, ensures that communication, sharing experience, best practice, and understanding the influence of other departments are improved. Most importantly, shared ownership of outcomes is included in the strategy implemented for optimizing results.

Leaders must ask themselves, "Does everyone have access to the education and training they need to be successful? Is leadership fueling personal and professional growth by creating a culture of ongoing learning?"

Education provided across teams with a common purpose also encourages trust. This increases team member confidence in the people they work with daily. Building trust is crucial to strengthening collaboration, delegation, team culture, and shared success. Education and training improve both performance and situational awareness. Common purpose and knowledge transcend the separation caused by silos and instead create an environment where people are engaged and driven to consistently put forth their best work—to be a part of something bigger than themselves.

Teams of Teams

When done correctly and consistently, education and training teach the learner how to increase performance; this is the essence of coaching, which is rare in healthcare systems. Physicians and nurses, as professionals, are imbued with a desire to provide the best care possible for their patients but often are confronted by policies, bureaucracy, documentation requirements, and functional silos that restrict their ability to optimize process flow. Adult learning structured as coaching can facilitate the creation of more effective teams, including teams that cross traditional operational departmental silos. These cross-functional teams—creating *teams of teams*—reduce conflict and ensure collaborative relationships, collaboration, and consensus instead of compromise.[21]

In 2012, I received a grant from the Vietnam Education Foundation through the United States Department of State to use education and simulation training to help teams (physicians, surgeons, and nurses) improve the ability to care for patients with kidney disease in Vietnam.[22] The idea was to improve process efficiency and to increase access to care. Partnering with Hue Medical School, we began with thirty-five students. The education and training included live interactive online sessions and three extended onsite programs emphasizing coaching and simulation-based team training. By the end of the eighteen-month training period, there were over 130 participants from across Vietnam. Teams developed an enhanced ability to provide care and significantly increased the number of patients receiving care, including dialysis and kidney transplantation.

There are many lessons learned from this experience. First, the power of adult learning, simulation training, and coaching was undeniable. The fact that social, language, and time zone barriers did not diminish the effectiveness impressed everyone involved. The emphasis on optimizing the ability of professionals to function at the highest level (top of license in today's terminology) was inseparable from the program's success. Incorporating high-reliability concepts and establishing the ultimate outcome measures as patient-centric ensured a common focus for all involved. People were brought together with a common purpose. This increased the success of people working together as teams, empowering them to optimize processes at the frontlines of patient care delivery.

In *Team of Teams: New Rules of Engagement in a Complex World*, General McChrystal and his co-authors describe how he transformed the slow-moving bureaucratic task force into an agile, adaptable network of teams united by a "shared consciousness," trust, and decentralized decision-making.[23] The strategies and accomplishments described in the book can be applied to healthcare. Changing management strategies to encourage and strengthen cross-functional teams reduces the negative influence of competition between operational silos. When working in teams, those on the frontlines experience improved adaptability and the ability to align resources with individual patient needs and manage risk and optimized outcomes more effectively.

The service line model used for certain complicated patient care, for example organ transplantation, shows the importance of a shared vision in delivering reliable quality care. Service lines are an example of the team of teams philosophy.

When examined closely, however, service lines are variable in their cohesiveness and independence. The influence of traditional departmental structures can be quite strong and reduce the availability of resources dedicated to the service line team over time. To be effective, the team must function as a unit to bring together people from different departments with complementary skill sets. Getting people from different departments together once a week or once a month for a meeting is not equivalent to working consistently as an established, empowered team sharing a vision of optimizing patient care.

Organizations should strive for transparency when it comes to decision-making processes. Making sure everyone understands the reasons behind decisions will help reduce the potential for misunderstandings between departments and encourage collaboration across the organization. Breaking down silos and encouraging collaboration between departments is essential for any organization that wants to remain competitive in today's market. Are your team members supported and properly positioned to do their best work? Empowering your people to shape their work and environments breeds a culture of engagement and accountability. Centralized micromanagement and "assembly line" mindsets inhibit the performance of professionals and the quality of their contributions. By taking steps such as fostering open communication, creating cross-functional teams, and promoting transparency in decision-making processes, organizations can create an environment where employees feel empowered and encouraged to work together towards common goals.

The complexity of the healthcare system means that additional changes are necessary to strengthen cross-functional team success. Some of these changes concern monetary policies upon which health systems rest—for example, aligning payment models with the team of teams concept in ways that optimize value. Optimizing care delivery and enhancing value can affect both resource utilization and revenue streams. For example, a team may decide that a patient would be better served by physical therapy than surgery after an injury. Applying complex system management strategies, such as establishing teams of teams, creates a common purpose, individually and collectively, that has a greater meaning beyond a specific specialty or volume target.

Breaking Down Silos

Complex healthcare systems must address departmental and budget silos to properly align process flow and ensure equitable access to quality patient care. This requires robust information sharing between departments. Data, especially in a raw form presented retrospectively, differs from what functional teams need when providing patient care. Healthcare teams need actionable information to aid in decision-making.

The inherent complexity of the healthcare system can, and most likely does, exceed the capacity of our ability to understand it fully. That is why advanced data analytics and accurate data analysis are necessary to make the most effective decisions. With patient health at stake, healthcare systems must have access to up-to-date information and powerful analytical tools to ensure patient safety and quality of care. The ability to understand risk at the individual patient level is important. Data analysis and actionable information can empower the frontline team to make more accurate and timely patient care decisions. Individualized patient information, ideally including physiologic, genetic, and socioeconomic information, facilitates prospective rather than reactive comprehensive care plans. With actionable information based on advanced data analysis, healthcare teams can make decisions more confidently and reduce costs by accurately aligning resources with needs. Cumulatively, the effect of increased information at the point of care delivery can help identify and manage risk, reduce error, and improve the patient experience.

Data analysis can also help healthcare providers better understand patient behaviors. Behavior has a large impact on health outcomes. Some experts estimate that patient behavior is responsible for at least 40 percent of patient care outcomes.[24] Patient behavior is challenging for healthcare teams to understand and impact. Patient self-reporting is often unreliable for various reasons, including embarrassment and lack of trust in the healthcare team. Advanced analytics can provide healthcare teams additional insight into factors influencing behaviors. This can lead to more accurate diagnoses and treatment plans tailored to individual patient needs.

The Butterfly Effect

The Butterfly Effect describes how small actions can cause significant changes over time and across silos in complex systems. This idea was first introduced by Edward Lorenz, a meteorologist, who noticed that even the most minor changes to a system's initial conditions could have drastic consequences on the weather.[25] Admittedly with hyperbole, he suggested that a butterfly's wings flap could cause a typhoon on the other side of the world.

Popular culture has embraced this concept, emphasizing the outsize significance of seemingly insignificant events or decisions. It also serves as an important reminder for leaders to be aware of how decisions in one area of a complex system can affect outcomes in unpredictable ways.

This principle has been applied to understanding patient outcomes within healthcare systems. A study conducted by The University of North Carolina School of Medicine found that small system-level changes can make a big difference in patient satisfaction and provide value-based care.[26] The authors concluded that patient care could be improved if the complexity of healthcare systems were better understood.

The butterfly effect reminds us that even small decisions can have far-reaching consequences and should not be taken lightly. To become more patient-centric and reliable, healthcare systems must accept complexity and employ strategies that improve process flow, minimizing disruption. If professionals at the frontline of patient care can recognize and respond rapidly to process flow disruptions, the impact of the butterfly effect can be minimized.

CHAPTER 6

MANAGING PROCESS WITHIN COMPLEXITY

"Out of intense complexities,
intense simplicities emerge."

WINSTON CHURCHILL

Process optimization is essential for high-reliability industries to become efficient and effective. It involves implementing structured methods, strategies, disciplines, and tactics to improve organizational processes. Process optimization aims to streamline operations, making it easier for teams to collaborate and complete tasks promptly. Organizations reduce or eliminate time and resource wastage, unnecessary costs, bottlenecks, and mistakes while improving efficiency. The goal is to make processes flow as efficiently and reliably as possible.

Process optimization begins by analyzing existing processes and identifying areas that need improvement.

> ## How to Analyze Existing Processes
>
> 1. Be clear and consistent about desired outcomes.
> 2. Beware of pre-existing bias.
> 3. Data needs to be timely and accurate.
> 4. Train team of teams to assess process flow and identify disruptions.
> 5. Consider simulation to test and evaluate process flow.
> 6. Process optimization requires a commitment to never being satisfied with the status quo.

Choosing the Primary Outcome

Analyzing process flow begins with defining the outcome of the process being evaluated. Truly defining the outcome is more complex than it might initially appear. We are predisposed to try to reduce complexity and devote our attention to isolated elements of the whole. W. Edwards Deming pointed out the potential error in relying on intermediary quality outcomes to demonstrate process success.[27] For example, a fire in a building can be put out rapidly, limiting the damage. People congratulate themselves for putting out the fire safely and might commit their resources to putting out fires. Putting out fires is important, but if that is our focus, what is done to fix the building and improve building codes to reduce the risk of subsequent fires? What have we done to identify and reduce risk?

Previously, we discussed how completing the checklist has become the measure of success in many hospitals instead of the improvements in patient outcomes the checklist is designed to support. Similarly, we might measure the time it takes to respond to a code blue alert in a hospital. We can easily calculate the time to respond, and we can conclude, rightfully, that patient lives are saved by a well-trained team getting to the bedside without unnecessary delay. A rapid response should certainly be celebrated. The problem is, if we stop there, what can we say about why patients require a code blue response?

If a patient comes to the hospital for an elective hip replacement, then has a respiratory arrest resulting in a code blue being called, the primary outcome measure should not stop with whether the code blue saved the patient's life. That is important to be sure, but the respiratory arrest is a flow disruption; an adverse outcome. From the perspective of future patients, the more significant outcome measure is decreasing the incidence of postoperative respiratory arrest. Risk needs to be identified and reduced.

As with the putting out fire example, the response time for a code blue alert measures the process itself, not the outcome of the process. More importantly, we need to understand the process flow disruptions that subjected the patient to increased risk and harm. Ultimately, the primary process outcome measures should align with patient-centric care goals.

The Impact of Bias

We all have biases. Bias occurs in various forms and presents in different ways. When speaking to physicians and nurses about patient safety and quality, I have often been told *they* have the sickest, most complicated patients. This bias reassures them they are doing their best under the circumstances and that any adverse outcomes are unavoidable. Similarly, someone will say they are the "only one" (presumably in the world) who can care for a specific type of patient or diagnosis. This might be true, but unlikely. If we accept the premise that patient care is delivered in a complex system, no one person or part of the system can stand in isolation if processes and resultant outcomes are optimized.

When assessing processes and outcomes with the goal of improvement, confirmation bias is important to recognize. Confirmation bias is the tendency to view information in a way that supports our pre-existing assumptions or views.

Surgery departments have the tradition of reviewing adverse outcomes, infection after surgery for example, in a meeting called Morbidity and Mortality (M&M). After reviewing a case, it is common that the conclusion is that "the complication was a known risk of surgery and was recognized and treated appropriately." At some level, this is an example of confirmation bias. The conclusion reassures the team that, given the circumstances, nothing different could have been expected or done. At least the response to the adverse outcome (process flow disruption) was timely and correct.

In this situation, the complexity of the system process that resulted in the infection may not be considered fully. Confirmation bias allows the analysis to stop when the information confirms what the team already believes to be true.

Biases, including confirmation bias, can be reinforced by experience. Personal preference is common, especially for physicians. How often has a student or resident been told to do something because the attending physician says, "That's the way I have always done it."

There is an adage that some doctors may not always be right, but they are never in doubt!

Learning and responding to circumstances where information is not complete forces us to take mental shortcuts (often incorporating past experiences and subject to bias). These mental shortcuts are called heuristics. They can speed decisions by skipping steps interpreted as unnecessary, but can lead to poor decisions due to limited data used to make decisions. An example would be ignoring a checklist because the physician's personal experience "proves" it does not make any difference. Consequently, risks are not recognized or appropriately managed, and process flow is not optimized.

In the context of complex system management, bias reduces the commitment to changing processes at a system level. Returning to our fire analogy, confirmational bias might reassure us that since we know wooden houses can burn, thankfully, we can put fires out. Our focus is on responding to a problem rather than preventing it.

Instead of spending most of our effort on putting out fires in healthcare, let's do more to prevent fires in the first place!

Actionable Information

To make sense of complexity, the ability of frontline caregivers to make timely and informed decisions is essential. In a simple, linear system where processes are highly repetitive and predictable, performance can rely on a combination of initial training reinforced by experience. Using intuition and heuristics to speed decision-making are usually effective in linear, highly predictable systems. However, as complexity increases, optimal human performance requires more in terms of support and alignment of resources.

Complex systems are never fully knowable, and interactions between system components are often unpredictable. As a result, people working at the point of patient care delivery must be supported in their ability to interpret and react to situations. Optimizing performance and achieving an optimal outcome, such as providing value-based care, requires making decisions in the context of the environment as it exists at the time. What is needed is to process, organize, and interpret the local situation? Professionals at the point of care delivery need information to empower them in decision-making.

What is the difference between information and data, and why is the distinction important? Physicians and nurses have access to a large amount of data, especially considering the modern electronic medical record. Data include a history of illness, previous notes documenting care, a list of medications, vital signs, etc. Data refers to unprocessed facts that may or may not be relevant to the current situation. Even if certain data are relevant, the importance of unprocessed raw facts is uncertain. Data requires organization and analysis to be useful to people needing to make decisions in complex systems.

When data is structured, analyzed, and presented in a meaningful and contextual way, it becomes information that can be acted upon. Information empowers people by supporting decision-making, increasing knowledge, understanding, and providing insights for specific purposes or goals. At the point of patient care, actionable information requires that the analysis not rely solely on historical, retrospective data. Relevance to the current situation is essential.

Information is the anecdote to reductionist attempts at oversimplification based on the assumption that complexity can be reduced to a linear construct. Information empowers people on the frontlines to move from rigid algorithms—step-by-step procedures—to processes incorporating individual circumstances and environmental realities to provide more effective patient-centric outcomes. Information guides the interpretation of variation at the patient level and reduces overly generalized assumptions. Regression to the "average patient" is at odds with the need to optimize performance in a complex, unpredictable environment.

Data refers to raw facts and figures, while information is the data processed to create a meaningful interpretation. Information facilitates understanding, decision-making, and knowledge acquisition. It provides relevance, context, and value.

Information can help to optimize human performance and empower people to make decisions. Information does not replace professional education, training, experience, and judgment. Instead, it supports and empowers. Today we have lots of data but little information. How can healthcare systems move from data to actionable information provided at the point of care delivery when needed?

Advancements in advanced analytics, such as machine learning (ML) and artificial intelligence (AI), are making their way rapidly into healthcare systems. ML and AI are technologies that enable machines to learn from data and make decisions without direct human intervention. Converting data to information that can be actionable in real-time could help healthcare teams choose optimal treatment paradigms and most effectively align resources to optimize patient outcomes. Automating these processes is key to success.

These technologies can help improve patient care by providing personalized treatment plans tailored to individual patients' needs. For example, AI-powered chatbots can provide 24/7 access to information about symptoms and treatments while helping patients manage their healthcare needs. It can automate tasks such as diagnosing medical conditions, analyzing medical images, and predicting patient outcomes.

For example, suppose a surgeon is seeing two patients with diabetes who have identical hernias. The patients have been sent to the surgeon by their primary care doctor to see about getting the hernias repaired. The surgeon informs the patients about hernia repair and discusses the risk of surgery. According to available information regarding risk, both patients are presumed to have the same risk based on being diabetic.

At this point, the surgeon has data (both patients would have the same surgical procedure, and both have diabetes) and the assumption is that both patients have the same risk of complications. The surgeon does not know actionable information to guide patient care in a way that optimizes care for these individual patients.

What would the impact on surgical risk be if the patients had very different socio-economic realities? Let us assume one patient lives in a wealthy suburb with many resources and strong family support. In contrast, the other patient lives alone in public housing without any family support or reliable transportation. Common sense tells us that the two patients have very different risk factors. Unfortunately, the reality is that today both these patients would almost certainly have the same pre- and post-operative care. Rather than having the information needed to understand and reduce the risk of adverse events, the healthcare team would be left to respond to any unexpected events or adverse outcomes.

Imagine if, instead, automated advanced risk analysis was done in real-time while the patient was being evaluated. This advanced risk analysis would include the diagnosis, medical history, socio-economic-related factors (social determinants of health), and perhaps even genetic information. The information that resulted from the data analysis would be presented to the healthcare team in real-time, detailing the individualized risk assessment and suggesting resources to mitigate any increased risk.

How could this information be used? A ride service to and from the hospital and clinic might be indicated for the patient without reliable transportation. Based on risk analysis and the resultant information, nutritional support and more frequent follow-up may be indicated. Automated analysis of data that provides actionable information improves the reliability of care by identifying and managing risk. In addition, resource allocation can be optimized by determining individual patient need. Providing resources based on an improved understanding of individual patient need and the benefit they will receive, reduces waste, and increases value. As we use information to improve the ability of healthcare teams to manage complexity, we can align resources more appropriately improving patient outcomes and patient satisfaction.

Another approach for moving from retrospective data to proactive information is robotic process automation (RPA). RPA is a type of software that automates routine tasks by mimicking the actions of humans.[28] It can automate administrative tasks such as scheduling appointments, processing insurance claims, and managing patient records. Automation technologies can improve process flow in healthcare, improving accuracy, increasing efficiency, and improving patient experience. By automating manual tasks with RPA, healthcare organizations can free up staff time for more important activities such as providing direct patient care. Automation can also help reduce errors caused by human error while ensuring compliance with regulations.

Other strategies include incorporating AI into telemedicine and remote patient monitoring to identify patient needs, some of which may otherwise not be recognized. Automated patient engagement tools incorporating advanced analytics can be used to optimize compliance with care pathways and facilitate additional support and resources to those at increased risk due to behavior, non-compliance, or other reasons.

Implementing these technologies in healthcare systems has challenges. AI requires significant resources to implement correctly. Advanced analytic systems must have access to large amounts of data to train and ensure high accuracy rates. Ensuring regulatory compliance when using automated systems is another challenge healthcare organizations face when utilizing AI, RPA, or remote patient monitoring technologies. Finally, healthcare organizations must be aware of the ethical implications of using AI and RPA technologies in healthcare, as these systems can potentially lead to bias or poor decision-making. Ideally, these tools should be designed and

implemented to provide information to the healthcare team to reinforce their knowledge, skill, and experience. By doing so, process flow
is optimized with a patient-centric focus.

Recognizing Disruption

Intuitively, most people recognize when a process is not flowing
smoothly. There may be interruptions, too many things competing
for attention, an inability to control the local environment, and poor
communication, which can result in frustration, anger, and burnout.
Recognizing disruptions in process flow can be more difficult in a
complex system because complex systems comprise multiple interdependent components that may be separated by distance and time.
Due to complexity, understanding how a process functions is only
partially knowable. Unexpected events and variability help to define
complexity. Nonetheless, there are strategies that teams can use to
assist in identifying process flow disruptions and identify solutions
to resolve them.

Direct observation is one way to assess process flow. Those observing processes must be trained and know the desired outcome. It is
possible to be confounded by intermediary process measures. Efforts
need to be in place to prevent that. Observers must select ways to
minimize the effect of pre-existing bias, especially confirmation bias.
A multidisciplinary observational team is ideal. It is also better if
those observing do not have pre-existing relationships with the people
doing the work, especially managerial or leadership relationships.

Observers should view the process from perspective of the patient.
By prioritizing the patient journey through the system being evaluated,
information is put in the context most relevant to patient outcomes
and experience. The time allocated for process observation must be
adequate to assess variability in the system.

Finally, observations are evaluated using both objective and subjective measures. Debriefing with the entire process team is important to ensure a comprehensive evaluation and transparency. During debriefing, data acquired by observation should be compared to related data obtained by other means, for example, from the medical record. When discrepancies are identified they need to be resolved.

Process flow disruptions can be identified using root cause analysis (RCA). RCA is a retrospective evaluation of factors believed to have contributed to an error. It has been applied successfully in many high-risk industries, including healthcare. The retrospective nature of RCA, as used in healthcare, means that pre-existing documentation and people's memory or recollection of events are the fundamental data elements from which conclusions are drawn. This imposes some limitations not present when using direct observation.

In healthcare, the results of an RCA are considered protected information, and consequently almost always remain within the confines of the hospital or facility where the RCA took place. Consequently, the information learned and the changes implemented as a result are rarely shared outside the facility where the RCA was performed. This contrasts with accident investigations done in other high-reliability organizations, such as the airline industry, where results of accident investigations are disseminated broadly.

Some years ago, we studied the application of simulation to evaluate errors and adverse outcomes.[29] In our study, RCAs that had been completed were replicated in a simulated environment. We found that participants identified system-level process flow disruptions not mentioned in the standard RCA. In addition, the team learned how people reacted to events in real-time and what knowledge, skill, and resources might have been used to prevent the error. In some cases, existing protocols restricted the simulation participants from acting to prevent an adverse outcome. They felt restrained by rules.

One example was the simulation of a patient who began bleeding after a procedure. In the actual case, the patient unfortunately died. In the RCA, the nurse was found to be at fault for not taking vital signs frequently enough. In the case simulation, the nurses participating consistently recognized what was happening and wanted to begin intravenous fluids to resuscitate the patient. However, the policy was that they needed a doctor's order, and given the circumstances, they could not contact a physician in time.

In addition to effectively identifying system process disruptions, our study demonstrated two important aspects of caring for patients within a complex system. First, the people at the frontlines of delivering care, the nurse in this example, need knowledge, training, and experience, coupled with resources and information. Most importantly, they need to be empowered to act to optimize patient outcomes. Overly restrictive policies, procedures, and rules that do not allow for judgment and being able to adapt to unexpected circumstances can create process flow disruptions that lead to error and potentially devastating adverse outcomes.

Second, the simulations reinforced the importance of establishing teams of teams. When managing a highly fluid, high-risk situation, the support of a multidisciplinary team increases situation awareness and the likelihood of a successful outcome. The simulation environment can be very effective in demonstrating the positive impact of teams of teams.

Complexity is Not Static

The simulation-RCA example illustrates the importance of responding to changing and unexpected situations. When applied to healthcare, one fallacy of linear system theory is that every situation can be anticipated, and the correct response known before the situation occurs. Complexity requires a different strategy, where control is decentralized and pushed to the point of care delivery. This does not mean there is no responsibility or accountability; the opposite is true. When frontline healthcare providers are empowered to make decisions, their professionalism and commitment increase. They begin to function more consistently at the "top of license," a place where knowledge, training, information, and resource utilization become essential. The responsibility of leadership is to provide the tools necessary for success.

Instead of asking, "What went wrong?" the question becomes, "What do you need for success?"

As empowerment and the resources to support it are increased, there is a heightened ability to understand process flow at the system level. Process flow optimization in complex healthcare systems is critical to providing quality patient care and managing costs. Process optimization involves identifying areas for improvement within existing processes and then implementing changes to increase efficiency, reduce waste, and improve outcomes. By optimizing processes, we can improve access, reduce disparities, improve patient satisfaction, reduce wait times, and maximize value.

Process optimization begins with an understanding of current pathways or healthcare processes. This includes sharing and analyzing data from different sources, such as patient records, billing information, operational metrics, patient outcomes, and direct observation. There are some things to keep in mind. One is that in complex environments, processes are not static but must be designed and managed to accommodate variability and the unexpected safely and reliably to avoid catastrophic failure. The patient's needs, and the patient's outcomes, must be put first when assessing process flow. The entire process and system must embrace quality as the performance metric that supersedes all others.

A few years ago, I established a team devoted to understanding process flow disruptions affecting patient care after surgery. The group was, in fact, a team of teams.[30] The team applied complex system management strategies to reduce disruptions and improve process flow. One significant accomplishment was a reduction in post-operative respiratory failure.

Post-operative respiratory failure (PORF) occurs when a patient unexpectedly needs to be intubated and placed on a ventilator after elective surgery. It is a publicly reported patient safety indicator. In evaluating process flow, the team of teams used several techniques. First, they conducted interviews. Interestingly, during the interview process they discovered that no one at the frontlines of patient care, including anesthesiologists, surgeons, intensivists, or nurses, knew the overall hospital rate of PORF. Uniformly, they were surprised that PORF occurred as frequently as it did. This lack of awareness is not uncommon in complex systems because of the independence of individual departments, even when functioning inter-dependently *from the patient's perspective*. Each operational unit, department, or individual provider might be aware of only two or three PORF events annually. From the individual perspective, PORF was uncommon, but that was not true at the system level when all cases were aggregated.

The team evaluated data related to PORF and identified risk factors. Then we began a period of observation of the surgical process. The observers were aware of known risk factors. At the end of the observation period, a diverse team discussed the findings and identified opportunities for process flow improvement.

A few of the most important results were unexpected. For example, room turnover time was a prominent performance metric for the operating room staff. There was administrative pressure to reduce the time between surgical patients. We identified that the constant emphasis on improving room turnover reduced the time allowed to extubate patients at the end of their surgery, contributing to PORF. This is an example of how emphasizing production targets can impact quality.

Another important process-related finding related to the drug Sugammadex. At the end of a surgical procedure, the anesthesiologist gives the patient medications to reverse paralysis, allowing them to breathe independently without a ventilator. Sugammadex is a new medication that is more expensive than older drugs that can be purchased as generic. Because Sugammadex is more expensive, the pharmacy department, and by extension the system, understandably wanted to carefully consider its use so as not to affect the budget adversely. A protocol was developed, in conjunction with anesthesiologists, that described "approved" patients who would potentially benefit most from the use of the more expensive drug. These included patients who were elderly and frail and prone to residual paralysis that might result in PORF.

The process observations and data review suggested that Sugammadex was rarely being used, even for the approved patients. The team carefully examined the process flow seeking a reason for the inconsistency in drug use. They discovered that the anesthesiologists were aware of the published data regarding the benefits of Sugammadex, so a lack of education was not the reason. Anesthesiologists were vocal in their opposition to restrictions that they felt undermined their professional judgment.

Ultimately, the investigation of process flow revealed that in addition to the guidelines for the use of Sugammadex, the pharmacy had taken the additional step of keeping the drug in the central hospital pharmacy instead of stocking it in the operating room area. This meant that if an anesthesiologist wanted to use the drug for a specific patient, they had to place an order electronically, then wait up to twenty minutes for it to be delivered. In part because of the emphasis on decreasing room turnover time, the anesthesiologists stated that it was not worth the effort or time required to obtain Sugammadex.

To resolve the process flow disruptions, the team arranged to have the drug stocked in the operating room to resolve this process flow disruption. In addition, the team provided additional education regarding PORF, the frequency it occurred, and the quality improvement initiative being implemented to improve patient outcomes. After six months of continuous quality improvement directed at process flow improvement, we demonstrated a 59 percent reduction in the incidence of postoperative respiratory failure.[31] The use of Sugammadex was increased but remained consistent with the approved guidelines. Not unexpectedly, the pharmacy budget was adversely impacted due to the increased use of the more expensive drug. However, when the cost of treating patients experiencing PORF was evaluated, the total cost of care decreased by more than $400,000, despite the increased cost of Sugammadex.

The quality improvement initiative to reduce postoperative respiratory failure illustrates that processes in a complex system have many components that interact, often in unexpected ways. This example also illustrates the importance of human behavior when considering complex system management. At the point of patient care delivery, professionals and teams can be restricted or empowered to provide optimal care. When patient care quality is the primary outcome measure for teams working within a complex system, conflicting priorities between silos can be resolved and collaboration optimized.

To achieve this goal, healthcare organizations must focus on continuous improvement by regularly assessing their processes and making necessary changes when needed. This cannot happen without appropriate resources, including knowledgeable professionals with time to commit to process improvement. An environment where staff feels empowered to suggest improvement ideas and collaborate with other departments is essential. Commitment includes resource allocation, such as expert leadership, time, and money. Allowing expert leaders to have time to be effective is an often neglected aspect of continuous quality improvement. Admittedly, this commitment can be expensive in terms of salary and other resources. Providing adequate time without other competing responsibilities is especially important. Meeting monthly at 6:30 a.m. for an hour is not an adequate commitment. The 6:30 a.m. meeting might check the box for "having a quality improvement committee," but from a practical perspective probably does not change much.

The return on investment of process flow improvement should be calculated from the total cost of care perspective. A challenge for healthcare organizations is that the ultimate beneficiary of cost savings may be the entity that pays for patient care. It is beyond the scope of this book to hypothesize about the need to consider alternative payment models. However, there is no doubt that in the complex healthcare system with many stakeholders, process optimization designed to provide the most effective patient care is inseparably intertwined with payment and the flow of money.

Process optimization is improving a process to make it more efficient and effective. Resolving flow disruptions and reducing risk requires analyzing existing processes to identify areas for improvement and then implementing changes that will optimize those processes.

The core principles of process optimization are:

1. Identify Process Flow Disruptions

   The first step in process optimization is identifying potential inefficiencies or bottlenecks in current processes. This can be done by analyzing data from previous iterations of the process and conducting interviews with stakeholders and employees who are familiar with the process. Observation, RCA, and simulation are tools to help identify flow disruptions.

2. Establishing Objectives

   Once disruptions have been identified, it's essential to set clear objectives for the optimization project. These objectives should be measurable and achievable, and they should also align with the overall goals of the organization. Patient-centric outcome measures should supersede process metrics.

3. Implementing changes

   After establishing objectives, it's time to start changing the process. This could involve introducing new technologies or tools, streamlining existing steps, or even wholly rethinking how specific tasks are performed. The plan-do-check-act (PDCA) cycle is a good method to support continuous quality improvement.

4. Measuring results

   Measuring the effect of changes made during the optimization process is essential to determine whether they are successful. This can be done by comparing data from before and after the implementation of changes and through feedback from stakeholders affected by the project. Patients must be included!

By following these principles of process optimization, organizations can ensure that their processes are running as efficiently and effectively as possible. It is important to think of process flow improvement as a continuous process. Since complex systems are variable and prone to unexpected events, process and quality improvement must be continuous. The team must believe that quality can always be improved. The PDCA cycle is a simple and well-known strategy that embodies a continuum of resolving process disruptions and managing change.[31]

Removing Waste

Resolving process flow disruptions is essential for improving value in healthcare systems by managing costs while simultaneously ensuring high-quality care is provided to patients. Everyday hospital and health system leadership is challenged by the waste in the system. Healthcare waste is a significant issue in the United States and worldwide. According to Brent C. James, MD, former chief quality officer of Intermountain Healthcare, approximately 30 percent of healthcare spending in the United States can be considered wasteful.[32] James outlines the importance of process flow optimization to reduce waste and improve patient outcomes. This includes unnecessary treatments, tests, and procedures that do not contribute to better patient outcomes. Implementing evidence-based practices, improving communication between providers and patients, and care coordination are examples of process flow improvement that can lead to significant cost savings. Important considerations include incorporating the principles of complex system management and avoiding the tendency to insist on reducing processes to a linear construct.

Oversimplification of processes can exacerbate disparities in patient care by imposing standards that do not accommodate socioeconomic status or other demographic characteristics that impact patient outcomes. Processes that are not optimized and do not adapt to individual patient needs contribute to higher levels of resource utilization.

Process flow improvements can help healthcare systems become more efficient and improve patient outcomes. By utilizing data collection and analysis tools and process redesign strategies, healthcare teams can reduce levels of waste while improving process flow and reliability in patient care. Process improvement can also help reduce disparities in care, leading to more equitable outcomes for all patients. With improved process flow and optimization, healthcare systems can become more efficient and cost-effective, ultimately leading to better health outcomes for all.

Complexity does not preclude process improvement. The opposite is true. Managing complexity requires continuous process improvement.

CHAPTER 7

CREATING RELIABILITY

"A man who lacks reliability is utterly useless."

CONFUCIUS

Process flow improvements are, in many ways, inseparable from high reliability. Many healthcare systems have pursued high-reliability concepts to improve accuracy and consistency. Much has been written about high-reliability organizations (HRO). Although differences in opinion exist regarding what elements define an HRO, a foundational element is avoidance of catastrophic failure. A preoccupation with failure is the most important aspect of HRO theory.[33]

At least in healthcare, a preoccupation with failure is challenging because it has, and continues to be, predominantly a responsive approach to something that already happened. Remember the example of putting out the house fire. If our attention is consumed with fixing problems rather than preventing them, how can we ever come out ahead?

We need to consider how a preoccupation with failure relates to optimizing quality, especially from the patient's perspective. A preoccupation with failure often assumes that errors and mistakes are unavoidable, and that reliability occurs when the ability to respond to an error, resilience, is built into the system. If we apply complex system management concepts, resilience is a given and the focus shifts to preventing error instead of responding to mistakes.

HRO philosophy can encourage a culture that emphasizes placing accountability (presumably for failures that will inevitably occur), which in practice is too often analogous to assigning blame. Finding the accountable person to blame may be satisfying on some level, since it provides closure, but it does nothing to address the process flow disruption that led to an error or adverse outcome. The role of leadership is to support processes that reduce the amount of risk people are exposed to while working within the system. Processes that anticipate and reduce risk will increase human performance, improve outcomes, and increase satisfaction.

A complex system approach empowers frontline professionals to use judgment, skill, information, and resources to optimize performance. This facilitates collaboration and coordination as a strategy to manage risk in real time and improve patient outcomes. By optimizing process flow, teams of teams can ensure that the right people are doing the right tasks at the right time, thus reducing errors and providing high-quality results. Process flow improvement helps organizations create uniform standards for process execution while avoiding limiting the ability to respond to changing circumstances.

Process flow optimization is crucial in allowing frontline workers to make the most appropriate decisions at the point of healthcare delivery. This allows them to quickly identify potential issues or areas of concern, enabling them to take corrective action before any problems arise. For frontline workers to make informed decisions, they need resources to be aligned, including access to accurate and up-to-date information. Process flow optimization helps ensure that appropriate resources are available and present in an easily accessible format and allocated most efficiently.

By streamlining workflows and eliminating unnecessary steps, process flow improvement can help teams of all sizes work more efficiently and effectively. One way process flow improvement can improve the function of teams is by breaking down complex tasks into smaller, more manageable chunks. This allows team members to focus on specific aspects of a project without getting overwhelmed or distracted by competing priorities.

Process flow optimization also allows for better collaboration between team members as everyone can be assigned the specific tasks they are best suited for. Team function is improved by identifying focus areas and prioritizing work accordingly. This ensures that team members are working on the most important tasks first while allowing them to delegate less important tasks or outsource them altogether.

Process flow improvement can help teams stay organized by creating clear task completion guidelines; checklists are an example. This can reduce process conflicts or confusion and ensure everyone is on the same page when completing projects or assignments. One important caveat is that organizations must incorporate and support regular education and training to empower teams to take full advantage of process improvement strategies. Complex system management requires those on the frontline to have the knowledge and skills necessary to perform at the highest level.

The best process flow improvements enable teams to become more agile in their approaches to patient care. Suppose a process needs to be updated based on new evidence, healthcare regulations, or industry trends. Continuous process flow improvement tools, like the PSCA cycle, can help identify what needs to be changed and how those changes should be implemented.

Overall, process flow improvement is invaluable for any

organization looking to increase team efficiency and productivity. By breaking down complex tasks into smaller chunks, identifying focus areas, and creating clear guidelines for completing tasks, process flow improvement can help teams work more effectively together, ensuring patient care is delivered efficiently without sacrificing quality.

Reducing Burnout

Process flow optimization can help mitigate burnout. No one will debate that burnout among medical staff is a growing problem in the healthcare industry.[34] It can lead to decreased patient satisfaction, impaired quality of care, and decreased productivity.

Many factors, including rigid standards and protocols, can cause burnout.[35] To reduce burnout, leaders should strive to create processes that allow physicians, nurses, and the entire frontline team appropriate autonomy (empowerment) to optimize patient care. Research suggests that rigid standards associated with linear process approaches can lead to burnout, especially if frontline employees feel their priority is not providing quality patient care. A study published in *The Joint Commission Journal on Quality and Patient Safety* found a correlation between burnout rates among doctors and increased administrative burdens.[36]

Improving process flow in healthcare systems can help reduce medical staff burnout by streamlining processes, reducing clerical tasks, and improving team functioning. This is especially true if the primary outcome measure is patient-centric and committed to the best patient experience. Process improvements can benefit medical staff by decreasing workloads and increasing job satisfaction. To facilitate process flow optimization, healthcare organizations should support their medical staff through initiatives such as regular feedback, positive reinforcement from supervisors, and reliable teams. By improving process flow in healthcare systems and supporting their medical team, healthcare organizations can reduce burnout while enhancing the quality of care for their patients.

Operations Management

Applying complex system management principles can seem daunting. Given healthcare systems' increasing scope and scale, managing day-to-day operations has many challenges. Short-term performance and damage control (putting out fires) can overwhelm the capacity of managers and leaders to consider comprehensive process optimization. The numerous operational silos that patients interface with further compound the difficulty of designing and implementing systems-level process approaches. To optimize process flow, there are a few critical solutions that managers and leaders should consider.

First, establish clear communication channels. Communication between team members is essential to be able to recognize and correct disruptions in process flow. Establishing communication channels and related protocols can help reduce the impact of disruption by allowing early goal-directed intervention.

It is important to acknowledge that effective communication is a learned skill. Communication is much more than being polite, although that certainly helps. Effective communication must be clear, concise, constructive, correct, and timely. Simply telling people they need to communicate is not enough. Teams must be taught how to communicate and practice the learned skills. Communication is a combination of speaking, listening, and non-verbal. Training is important to help team members understand their communication style's impact on others, both positive and negative, and how it might be improved. As with all process design and optimization components, the objective is to improve patient care reliability, safety, and value. A commitment to effective communication is inseparable from achieving these goals.

Effective communication supports and reinforces team performance and situational awareness. It builds trust. Trust is strengthened by shared learning and training, empowerment, collaboration, and compassion. Effective communication between team members reinforces effective processes and facilitates corrective action when processes need to be adapted to changing situations. Tools that support process flow, such as checklists, cannot perform as designed without effective communication.

Second, ensure that those metrics are consistent with the process output (patient outcome) and not the process itself. Monitoring throughput, cycle time, and quality metrics can help identify areas at greatest risk for process flow disruption. This data can then be used to adjust and improve the process flow. Predictive analytics can anticipate potential problems before they occur, allowing operations managers to take proactive steps to prevent or mitigate them before they become disruptive. The goal should be to identify weakness in processes and correct them before they adversely impact patient care. Predictive models incorporating patient information such as physiologic, genetic, and socio-economic can identify and even predict process flow disruptions and the associated risks.

AI and ML have the potential to revolutionize process flow by allowing for more accurate diagnoses, treatments, and procedures. AI can automate specific processes, thus reducing the disruptions caused by manual intervention and ensuring that workflow is consistent. AI can also be used to identify areas of disruption in the process flow and suggest solutions to improve efficiency.

AI and ML can improve process flow by optimizing patient care and reducing errors due to misdiagnoses or by suggesting optimized treatment pathways. It can also detect risks associated with treatments and provide timely warnings of any potential complications. By providing data-driven insights into complex processes, effectively incorporating advanced analytics in complex system management can transform healthcare delivery systems by improving the speed and accuracy of diagnoses while reducing waste. Overall, AI and ML have the potential to revolutionize process flow in healthcare settings by speeding up diagnoses, reducing human error, optimizing patient care, and improving overall efficiency.

Reliability Requires People

As process flow improves, teams can work more efficiently and effectively. Cohesive teams can manage complexity by breaking down complex tasks into smaller, more manageable chunks and identifying focus areas to prioritize. This cannot occur without effective communication, which is a foundational element of team performance in a complex environment. Complex system management depends upon improving the function of individuals and "teams of teams"—to work together towards common goals or objectives—patient-centric care and the best possible patient experience.

Well-designed processes help organizations create uniform expectations for process execution. This allows all team members to be on the same page and ensures everyone follows procedures correctly. When optimized, process flow enables teams to become more agile in their approaches by allowing them to adopt new processes or adjust existing ones as needed to individualize patient care. By leveraging process flow improvement tools, healthcare organizations can improve patient care while meeting ever-changing demands.

Another way process flow optimization can benefit frontline workers is by assisting them to become more engaged in their work, reducing frustration and burnout. By providing them access to automated processes, they can focus on tasks that require their expertise instead of spending time on mundane tasks such as paperwork or data entry. This allows them to be more productive and efficient, which ultimately leads to better decision-making at the point of healthcare delivery.

Process flow optimization can also help improve communication between frontline employees and various organizational departments. Streamlining processes and ensuring everyone has access to the same information makes it easier for different departments within an organization to collaborate and share resources when needed. This helps ensure that everyone involved in a particular decision-making process has all the necessary information to make the best possible decision for their patients.

Empowerment

Empowering frontline healthcare workers is at the core of complex system management. Empowering people to function at the top of their license—applying knowledge, skill, and judgment—during every patient encounter is necessary to optimize processes for high reliability. There are many reasons for this. Processes that manage complexity by decentralizing control engage team members more than rigid, inflexible, centralized processes. Frontline workers have the most direct contact with patients, and therefore are well-positioned to make decisions that best meet the needs of each patient.

Optimized processes support team members directly engaged in patient care, allowing them to respond quickly and efficiently to individual patient needs, including when the unexpected occurs. Resources can be more effectively aligned with needs. Promoting the team of teams construct is a form of empowerment that can help by allowing frontline team members to make informed decisions.

Patient satisfaction improves with provider team empowerment, which enables frontline employees to respond more compassionately to patient concerns and unique circumstances. Processes that include effective communication further increase trust between patients and their care providers, because they feel like their concerns are being heard and taken seriously.

Empowerment can also reduce factors associated with burnout by increasing job satisfaction among frontline team members, who feel trusted and valued for their expertise and experience. Processes that are effective in a complex environment not only empower team members but provide the structure enabling them to function at the highest level, helping to ensure that healthcare organizations remain competitive in an increasingly complex healthcare landscape.

CHAPTER 8

VARIABILITY

"Variability is the law of life, and as no two faces are the same,
so no two bodies are alike, and no two individuals react alike and
behave alike under the abnormal conditions which
we know as disease."

WILLIAM OSLER

In the latter half of the twentieth century, advances in medical and surgical care began happening at an explosive rate. Procedures like organ transplantation, which had been science fiction, have become common. Our ability to care for older and sicker patients has created an atmosphere of invincibility as healthcare teams push the limits of what can be done. There are amazing stories of success, of saving lives, some of which are truly heroic. However, results (patient outcomes) are inconsistent, and the reasons are unclear.

There are those who believe the physician's knowledge and skill is the ultimate determinant of success, but data did not support this hypothesis. Studies have looked at surgeon volume to determine if there is a direct correlation with patient outcomes. That intuitively makes sense. If someone does more of something, they should be better. However, this is not consistently true. Some surgeons have high volumes but poor results; the opposite is also true. Some surgeons do a relatively small number of highly specialized surgeries with excellent results. Hospital outcome data is similarly difficult to interpret. For example, some hospitals have experienced improved outcomes when experienced surgeons leave and new surgeons are added to the team.

How can these data related to professional performance and patient outcomes be resolved? How can variable patient outcomes become more consistent? What process strategies can be used to manage the inevitable variability in a complex system?

Enhanced Recovery

To reduce variability in surgical outcomes, surgeons began to investigate what aspects of the surgical care process—the patient journey—were associated with the best patient outcomes. As research and data sharing progressed, processes associated with more consistent results were identified. For example, having the patients shower the night before surgery, giving antibiotics before the skin incision was made, using a pre-surgical checklist, starting nutrition sooner after surgery, and getting patients up and walking. These process components are surprisingly simple but were recognized as inconsistently used for patient care.

The surgeons advocating for process improvement argued that if the elements of best practice could be incorporated into an optimized process that could be replicated widely, then patient outcomes would be improved and variability reduced. A concerted effort to accomplish this began in Europe in the late 1990s.

Enhanced Recovery After Surgery (ERAS), also known as fast-track surgery or enhanced surgical recovery, results from this innovative work to improve surgical patient care processes. The concept of ERAS was pioneered by a group of surgeons led by Prof. Henrik Kehlet from Denmark.[37] In the late 1990s, Kehlet and his colleagues challenged the traditional paradigm of prolonged fasting, bed rest, and restrictive perioperative practices. They recognized that such practices led to increased patient discomfort, prolonged hospital stays, and higher rates of complications. Kehlet proposed a paradigm shift towards a more patient-centered approach emphasizing early mobilization, optimized pain control, and judicious fluid management.

ERAS is a process that empowers multidisciplinary teams to optimize the entire surgical journey and improve patient outcomes. The process involves a set of evidence-based protocols and interventions implemented before, during, and after surgery to minimize surgical stress, enhance recovery, and reduce postoperative complications. The impact of ERAS on patient care has been significant.

The initial efforts to implement ERAS focused primarily on colorectal surgery. In 2001, Kehlet and colleagues published a landmark study demonstrating the benefits of ERAS protocols in colorectal surgery.[38] The study showed significant reductions in postoperative complications, length of hospital stays, and costs without compromising patient safety. This study laid the foundation for the widespread adoption of ERAS principles in various surgical specialties.

Since then, ERAS programs have been developed and refined for a wide range of surgical procedures, including orthopedic, gynecologic, urologic, and thoracic surgeries. These programs involve a collaborative effort among surgeons, anesthesiologists, nurses, physiotherapists, and other healthcare professionals to implement evidence-based interventions tailored to each surgical specialty.

The impact of ERAS on patient care has been remarkable.

Numerous studies have demonstrated that processes incorporating ERAS principles significantly improve patient outcomes. Improved outcomes include reduced rates of surgical site infections, ileus (time to be able to eat after surgery), urinary tract infections, pulmonary complications, and overall mortality. ERAS-based process flow improvements have also been associated with shorter hospital stays, faster recovery of gastrointestinal function, earlier return to normal activities, and improved quality of life for patients. Not unexpectedly, improvements in process and patient-centric outcomes resulting from ERAS has demonstrated cost-effectiveness by reducing healthcare resource utilization and overall healthcare costs.

The success of ERAS is an example of successful process optimization. ERAS does not restrict healthcare teams. Instead, the resulting process optimization empowers teams to perform at a higher level. Well-designed processes do not fail when confronting variability, they improve the ability of the team to respond effectively.

The history of enhanced recovery after surgery has seen a paradigm shift in perioperative care, applying a process flow that impacts the entire patient journey. This does not mean that every patient is the same, but rather every patient deserves a baseline standard of care based on evidence associated with the best patient-centric outcomes. By challenging traditional practices and implementing evidence-based protocols, ERAS has revolutionized patient care across various surgical specialties.

ERAS is most effective when multiple elements are incorporated into a comprehensive process. Applying complex system theory, we recognize that the various elements are interdependent and interact in ways that are not always predictable or even fully knowable. If we try to pull apart the individual components of an ERAS protocol and assign a predictable contribution or outcome associated with each element (a reductionist, linear approach), the benefits begin to diminish. The remarkable thing about ERAS is that it begins by accepting complexity and then manages uncertainty by establishing standard processes that the frontline healthcare team can adapt to individual circumstances.

Complexity and Variability

Complexity is variable, and variability is complex. The two are inseparable. We can ignore this and try to reduce complexity to a simple-to-understand linear construct, but that will never reflect reality, especially for healthcare. We are faced with the challenge of creating processes that allow us to respond to variability while ensuring that patient outcomes are equitable and consistent. Processes must be designed and implemented to ensure the value of healthcare is maximized.

Healthcare variability manifests in many ways, including inconsistent care practices, poor outcomes, and excessive costs. ERAS is a successful approach to reducing the negative impacts of variability on patient outcomes. Experts have argued that healthcare variability must be reduced to control costs and improve care. Still, the promise of the effort to reduce variability has yet to deliver the promised results consistently. Healthcare costs keep rising, and overall patient outcomes have not improved.

As a patient, we want assurance that we are receiving appropriate, evidence-based healthcare tailored to us as individuals to have the best potential outcome. That is not the same as wanting our healthcare to be standardized to the point that the exact same treatment is prescribed to every patient every time. As Osler accurately pointed out more than one hundred years ago, no two individuals experience healthcare the same way.

If we accept that healthcare is provided in a complex environment, then the assumptions and processes we work with must function reliably, even under conditions of uncertainty. Further, if our objective is to simultaneously optimize patient outcomes, to be reliable, and to provide value, then we must manage complexity because we cannot control it. Managing and reducing the impact of variability cannot be equated to eliminating variability by imposing rigid standards and overly simplified linear processes. Processes enabling professionals to function in a complex environment do so by supporting, not overly restricting. Optimized processes create a culture that encourages people and teams to perform at the highest level possible.

In managing complexity, accountability and blame transform into empowerment. Reacting to error and adverse outcomes is converted to continuous quality improvement. Instead of focusing on putting out fires, attention is directed to prospectively assessing risk, optimizing processes, and improving resource allocation in ways that result in the best patient outcomes. Expecting people to follow immutable rules (of which there are too many ever to remember) becomes optimizing performance using knowledge, training, information, and resource alignment. Instead of creating work environments where people are forced to be individually responsible, teams offer support and backup.

Processes must be responsible and adaptable, or else complexity and variability will be unmanageable, leading to inconsistent and unacceptable outcomes.

Consequences

Small decisions can have far-reaching consequences in healthcare systems, significantly affecting patient care. Due to the system's inherent complexity, deciding between treatment options can be daunting for both patients and clinical teams. For example, when patients face too many choices, they may be unable to decide and risk not receiving the best care. Patients may experience gaps or fragmentation in care as they try to navigate the system. They may receive inconsistent and conflicting healthcare advice. Healthcare providers may be forced to make decisions based on incomplete knowledge or anecdotal data, leading to inaccurate diagnoses or treatments. Complexity can interfere with communication and trust. As a result, the patient-provider relationship may be strained, lacking compassion. Ideally, processes designed to work in a complex environment should encourage shared decision-making between patients and healthcare providers.

Healthcare systems must recognize the importance of decisions related to process design to ensure that patients receive the best possible care and experience. Healthcare providers must be aware of the potential consequences of how small choices might disrupt process flow and take steps to reduce the associated risk. This includes effective communication and evidence-based processes supported by actionable information, enhancing the ability to make informed decisions. The best processes encourage shared decision-making between patients and providers.

Emphasizing eliminating variability as a core priority conflicts with the realities of working within a complex system. There are many reasons for variability that cannot be modified but must instead be accommodated. For example, variability in healthcare can arise from differences in patient characteristics that we cannot control, such as genetics, past medical history, stage of disease at presentation, and social determinants of health. Patients are not the only source of variability. Variability is also present in the local healthcare environment. Provider skill, training and experience, the availability of resources, and even the time of day all contribute to variability.

By accepting that variability exists, we can develop processes to manage it effectively instead of devoting time and energy to futile attempts at elimination or control.

One approach to managing variability is to empower professionals to use their judgment and expertise to optimize patient care by implementing processes that are flexible. This approach is more rational than trying to eliminate variability using rigid top-down control. This is not to say that there are not standards of patient care; quite the opposite. Processes designed to be effective in a variable environment must be firmly grounded by standards and guided by evidence.

For example, there is evidence that some procedures, like knee replacements, can be done safely and effectively as an outpatient if specific processes are followed. Research has shown that when knee replacement is done as an outpatient, costs are reduced, patient outcomes are equivalent or even improved, and patient satisfaction is increased.[39] However, assuming all patients are suitable for outpatient total joint replacement can lead to adverse outcomes. A patient may have a chronic disease requiring blood thinners or inadequate family support at home. There will be patients who cannot be safely managed using standard outpatient care pathways without additional support. The process can promote outpatient surgery while ensuring reliable, high-quality outcomes by adapting to individual patient realities.

When managing patient variability, the healthcare team should be empowered to make critical decisions that minimize process flow disruptions. Understanding and predicting individual patient resource needs and aligning resources appropriately is necessary. A highly standardized assembly line approach that does not accommodate variability can exacerbate disparities, resulting in avoidable cost and frustration for both the healthcare team and the patient.

It is important to consider factors such as patient preferences and individual circumstances to reduce variation in care quality. A one-size-fits-all approach is not always appropriate or effective. Instead, healthcare providers should strive to provide care tailored to each patient's unique needs and preferences. To ensure that processes are effective in a complex system, leaders should find ways to encourage creativity and innovation while still adhering to established standards. Appropriately responding to variability is simplified when the outcome priority is clearly, consistently communicated and adhered to.

Leaders can tailor their approach when using best practices in complex systems by understanding two major lessons of complex systems. The first lesson is that small events can lead to significant challenges, meaning that organizations should be aware of potential risks and plan accordingly. The second lesson is that you can't predict if attempts to improve things will work, so leaders must be prepared for unexpected outcomes and have a plan for dealing with them. By incorporating the ability to respond to specific needs when designing and implementing processes, teams are effectively supported in their efforts to achieve optimal patient care.

Constant monitoring of outcomes and the variables encountered in delivering care is essential. Relying on retrospective nonclinical data, such as billing data, is inadequate. To optimize and continually improve processes, analytic expertise is needed to understand how processes are functioning and where disruptions are or are likely to occur. The risk of process flow disruption needs to be constantly assessed and prospectively addressed.

When Variability Doesn't Matter

When we get on a commercial airliner, we don't ask who the pilot is or where they went to school. We don't question whether the maintenance team is better at United or Delta or Southwest. We are confident that best practices are maintained, not just for one company but across the industry. The commitment to high reliability and safety reassures us that variability in core processes is minimized. Because safety is the highest priority outcome, and information is shared transparency, we assume that the knowledge and training are equivalent, irrespective of the airline. The record of safety reassures us that fundamental processes are consistent across the commercial aviation system.

At the same time, this level of consistency or standardization does not mean that professional judgment and adaptability to variable circumstances are eliminated. Instead, the team-oriented culture of safety mandates that situational awareness, effective communication, regular training, and the ability to react appropriately to changing circumstances be supported. For example, let's consider how the approach to potentially dangerous weather has evolved.

The unpredictability of weather affects many high-reliability organizations. Examining how the airline industry manages risk related to weather, we see an evolution that can be roughly divided into three periods. As the jet age began to flourish, there was confidence that the pilots' skill and the aircrafts' strength could safely manage any weather. The processes emphasized the independence of the pilots to make decisions. They were the captains of the ships, after all. At the time, most pilots had come from the military and had excellent training and many hours of flight time. Many were combat-decorated heroes.

Unfortunately, the processes followed during this era did not always emphasize safety as the ultimate outcome measure of success. Intermediary process measures, like on-time arrival, were at times prioritized. Processes at the time permitted pilots to fly through bad weather on takeoff or landing, confident in their skill and the aircraft. As a result, the accident rate was unacceptably high, especially by today's standards.

This is analogous in many ways to healthcare and surgery today.

There are "Top Gun" contests for surgeons and frequent positive comparisons to fighter pilots. Taking risks is assumed to equate to saving lives. For many, the surgeon remains the ship's captain, bearing all responsibility. If processes do not prospectively manage risk, too many adverse outcomes are the result. Simply identifying risk in a complex system does little to improve reliability, safety, or outcomes. Risk needs to be identified and processes adjusted to reduce the possibility of an adverse outcome.

In the second era, avoiding landing in a storm became a priority. More was known about the risks associated with severe storms, including microbursts. A significant process change was to fill the airplane with extra fuel so that it could circle, sometimes for hours, if there was adverse weather at the arrival airport. Waiting for the weather to improve prior to landing reduced accidents, but at a significant cost in time and fuel.

We can think of similar situations in healthcare where our approach to risk management is to order unnecessary tests or procedures. These processes may reduce the occurrence of some adverse outcomes, but they increase waste and cost without a clear correlation with improved outcomes.

Today, the pilots and crews are supported by a sophisticated system that can predict the weather at the arrival airport many hours in the future. We have all experienced pulling away from the gate and then waiting on the tarmac for a departure time. In this process flow, the pilot's judgment and skill is supported by information and effective communication. The process design acknowledges that there will be variability and has identified the safest, most cost-effective way to manage it. We, as passengers, trust that the pilot is using a combination of their training, skill, and judgment, supported by a system that works together to keep us safe.

In contrast to the airline pilot example, process variability in healthcare continues to affect patient outcomes by introducing discrepancies between treatments received from different providers. Even in the same hospital, there can be significant differences in care approaches. In some cases, this could mean that a patient receives a lower quality of care than they should. Process design should emphasize patient outcomes as the goal and empower providers in real-time to optimally use judgment, skill, appropriate resources, and information. The system needs to support the processes, and the processes need to support the frontline worker.

Alignment

To optimize performance in a complex system, we must simultaneously manage variability by establishing standards aligned with and supporting the highest quality outcomes. At the same time, process design must ensure that human performance is not impaired by rigid rules that cannot accommodate individual patient or situational variability. Balancing these objectives begins with understanding where processes can manage variability and uncertainty.

Complexity forces us to think and act in new ways. The complexity of a large organization is increased by silos and misaligned performance metrics, as we have discussed. If individuals within a complex system only focus on their own department's performance goals, achieving the best patient outcome is difficult, if not impossible. It might be human nature but working to maintain the status quo within one departmental silo will restrict innovative process design or implementation. As healthcare leaders develop strategies to manage complexity, a resolute commitment to optimizing patient-centric outcomes and value provides the solid foundation for the system's culture. In this commitment, we can respond to and manage variability without futile attempts to control complexity.

Studies have shown that variability in healthcare can lead to increased costs and poorer patient outcomes.[40] Unmanaged variability can negatively affect patient outcomes and increase waste and cost. Healthcare organizations should strive to optimize processes to increase the reliability of achieving high-quality, patient-centric outcomes. This requires a system-level approach. It begins with focusing on patient quality outcomes that supersede other process performance measures.

Education and Training

Organizations must commit to continued education and training as part of the strategy to manage complexity. Ongoing and meaningful training that includes simulation is an important component of most high-reliability organizations. Unfortunately, this is not true in healthcare. The structure of professional specialization and licensing means that there is little consistency in the information learned or how current the knowledge is. The current continuing medical education (CME) structure is designed to achieve competency—having essential knowledge and skills. To optimize processes in a complex system, we need to strive for proficiency—the mastery of skills.

There is value in specialty-specific ongoing education to be sure. Unfortunately, CME is almost always provided exclusively to the individual. The team working together is unlikely to learn or train together. This limitation can be overcome, to a degree, by creating a team of teams where individual expertise and knowledge come together to contribute to improving the team's functional capability. However, to perform at the highest level, team members need to spend time learning and training together. Only in that way will teams be more prepared to function effectively in a complex environment.

Imagine a professional football team. What if education and training were designed so that each member or specialty of the team trained separately? The quarterback trains separately from the running back, and the offensive line is separated from the running backs. They train hard each day, but always separately, never practicing together. Each may be competent as individuals, but is there any way the team can be proficient? Then the team members come together on Sunday to play a televised game. How would that turn out?

This football example is far-fetched. No professional or amateur team would be coached that way, but that is what happens daily on the frontline of healthcare. The patient care team members almost always learn and train in isolation, sometimes receiving conflicting information, then are put together to care for patients, including the most complicated cases. Amazingly, it usually works, but not always, contributing to adverse outcomes, avoidable deaths, and waste. Not to mention the contribution to frustration and burnout.

Managing complexity must include the health system leaders supporting education and training. Expertise, time, and resources need to be committed. Expertise in adult education and simulation is needed, as is the time away from clinical activity to take advantage of their expertise. Essential ongoing education supporting professional development in areas like situational awareness, teamwork, and communication are ways to empower professionals to perform at the highest level possible. Ensuring that team members have the knowledge to contribute to process development and continuous improvement is a bottom-up, decentralized approach to help manage complexity.

We must increase our commitment to ensuring that healthcare team members are well-informed about evidence-based care, the use of best practices, and how to respond effectively when unforeseen circumstances arise (situational awareness). Continual education and training are foundational to coping with complexity and managing the associated variability. Education also helps establish a safety and reliability culture by demonstrating how we all contribute to success or to failure.

Silos Contribute to Variability

Authors such as Michael E. Porter have written extensively about the importance of reducing variability in healthcare to improve patient outcomes and reduce waste and costs. Porter argues that variability needs to be significantly reduced to reduce overall healthcare costs.[41] Similarly, Atul Gawande has argued that standardizing protocols across healthcare organizations can lead to better patient outcomes by reducing variability in care.[42]

As we develop strategies to manage variability, we must consider the interdependency of operational units or silos within the system. Ideally, our perspective must be from the patient's; we can only align processes with patient-centric outcomes. The consequences of processes in one silo must not adversely affect the function and flow of processes in another. To achieve consistency, the silos must not have competing performance metrics. Departments need to support each other and be interdependent, not independent. Processes need to ensure that individual department efforts are coordinated and working toward a common goal.

In today's complex healthcare systems, processes within different departments may not be coordinated. The resulting variability in process flow can make defining value difficult and reduce patient satisfaction. Lack of alignment, including with respect to performance metrics, can create poor quality outcomes such as delays in care, errors in patient records, or even unnecessary procedures. Using key performance indicators (KPIs) to measure the effectiveness of patient care within a complex healthcare system can have unintended consequences. While KPIs are essential for providing guidance and direction for managers, if they become too narrowly focused on individual goals, they can lead to process flow disruptions that negatively impact patient outcomes. If KPIs are not aligned with patient care experiences across the system, this variability in process flow will be perpetuated instead of addressed.

For example, one department might focus solely on efficiency by reducing patient visits. At the same time, another department might believe more frequent patient visits prevent hospital admissions. Some patients may have care that occurs in both departments and consequently receive contradictory information regarding how often they need to be seen. Communication breaks down without proper alignment of process goals across different system areas, and patient care experiences become fragmented. It is essential for leaders to carefully consider how KPIs are used to measure success and guide managers. Aligning KPIs with patient care experiences across the entire system will ensure that patient safety remains paramount so that cost savings are achieved without impacting the quality of service and the greatest value is derived.

Data, Analytics, and Information

When information can be delivered to the frontline healthcare team in real-time, they can further improve process flow and optimize patient care. Rather than relying upon published information that might not be relevant to a specific patient, new innovative technology allows evidence-based processes to appropriately accommodate the variability encountered on the front line of care delivery. Imagine a more effective alignment of resources with individual patient need, supported by information. Aligning resources can effectively reduce risk, waste, and error. AI and ML have the potential to support healthcare providers to optimize safety and value, the same way air-traffic control tells pilots to wait for take-off because bad weather is predicted in the future at the time of landing.

By monitoring patient satisfaction scores or patient outcomes over time, organizations can gain insight into what processes are working well and which need to be adjusted or improved. The challenge is to keep the focus on patient-centric quality performance targets. Those responsible for applying data analytics must avoid the tendency to use data to find out what was done wrong. Instead, the optimal use of data is to improve processes to maximize quality throughout the patient care process.

Transformative change will occur when data shifts from retrospective to prospective and is provided to the patient care team as actionable information to help optimize patient care in real-time. To be useful, information, in addition to being available at the point of care delivery, must help the care team provide individualized care given the resources available. By providing information when needed to optimize process flow and team performance, data analytics can ensure that patients receive reliable, high-quality care.

CHAPTER 9

COMPASSIONATE ACTION

"True happiness comes from a sense of inner peace and contentment, which in turn must be achieved through the cultivation of altruism, of love and compassion and elimination of ignorance, selfishness, and greed."

THE DALAI LAMA

At this point, I hope you agree that healthcare occurs in a complex system! You might be thinking, "Since it is so complex, there is nothing I, as an individual, can do. Some of the smartest people in the world have been working on this, yet costs keep rising, disparities in care do not seem to be any better, and there continue to be errors and avoidable deaths."

All that is true, but still, as individuals, we can be part of the solution. A commitment to optimizing processes in a way that empowers people to provide the best possible patient care is a great place to start.

People choose a career in healthcare to have a positive human impact and to make a difference. Leadership and management are responsible for establishing, optimizing, and being committed to processes that empower the healthcare team to "do the right thing, for the right patient, at the right time."

Admittedly, there are many layers to the healthcare system—that is part of its complexity! This book purposefully does not cover topics such as the insurance/payor system, employed vs. private practice physician models, the influence of government, or the impact of tort law and medical malpractice. My objective is to provide a framework that can be used to design and implement processes that help manage complexity and in doing so increase reliability, improve safety, and manage cost. Ultimately, processes designed to work with instead of in opposition to complexity will improve patient-centric outcomes. Both patients and healthcare teams will have greater satisfaction if the processes are more efficient, less frustrating, and provide better outcomes.

Where to Start

*A place to start is to consider that at some point,
each of us will be a caregiver and, at some point, a patient.*

This truth reminds us that the path to healthcare improvement requires understanding the perspectives of all involved. There will be different perspectives, and priorities might not always align. We must be compassionate to work together and find common ground in creating processes that lead to patient-centric improvement.

Unlike empathy, compassion responds to another person's struggles with a sincere desire to help. Leaders responsible for creating a positive culture in a complex environment are most effective if they are compassionate. We have discussed how complex system management requires decentralization and empowering people and teams. A self-serving leader who sees control as essential to maintaining their position will not effectively champion processes designed to optimize performance at the point of care delivery.[43]

We have discussed the advantages of a "team of teams" when working within complex environments and managing variability and uncertainty. Compassion is essential for teams to function effectively. Effective communication, collaboration, interpersonal trust, and an appreciation for the contributions of others are all consistent with showing compassion. Compassion empowers team members to support each other and collectively provide the best possible care.[44]

Health is central to humanity. We all have the right to protect and improve our health as individuals and collectively. The healthcare system must respond compassionately to the healthcare needs of the individuals and populations served.

The complexity of our healthcare system can obscure compassion, especially from the patient's perspective. To be effective, processes must rest upon a foundation of compassion. The strategies presented in this book to improve process flow rest upon a compassionate vision of optimizing care for fellow human beings. Without compassion, any actions we take will not be effective and may, in fact, cause harm. If our process improvement efforts rest firmly on a foundation of compassion, then the nuances of managing complexity become evident. Compassion compels us to manage complexity in healthcare designing and using processes that do the right thing for our patients and for those we work with.

Compassion, emphasizing serving others, helps us align purpose, establish trust, and commit to improving patient care.

Start Small

Process improvement can be accomplished by applying complex system management strategies. At the same time, our understanding of complexity reminds us that we can never fully control the system. Leaders can begin the process by educating team members about complexity and sharing strategies for managing it. Advocating for patient-centric outcomes consistently being the primary objective is the most compelling place to start.

The next step is to create teams of teams charged with improving processes within their sphere of influence. Leaders and teams can then incorporate the Ten Core Principles for Complex System Process Management in Healthcare. Effective, transformative change takes vision and commitment. It is a continuous process that must adapt to an ever-changing environment. Most importantly, people are the process—whether working to improve processes, working within a process, or, especially as a patient, being affected by the process and its flow.

Processes alone cannot manage complexity; they help guide people aspiring to provide the best care possible for their patients. Ultimately, inspiration, innovation, and compassion will help you manage complexity using processes that empower people to do the right thing for the right patient at the right time.

Ten Core Principles for
Complex System Process Management in Healthcare

1. Ensure that patient-centric quality outcomes are the primary measure of success. As process design and implementation advance, leaders and team members must ensure that the focus on the outcome of the process, not the process itself.

2. Embrace complexity. Design processes that are responsive and adaptable. Optimizing performance includes being able to respond to the unexpected. Leaders and all involved

must resist the temptation to reduce every process to an overly simplified, linear construct.

3. Create and empower teams of teams. The work of process optimization is best done by people who have the most knowledge. By decentralizing process design and implementation, the effectiveness of a process can be interpreted in real-time.

    * *Leaders must give team members the tools they need to succeed. Accountability becomes "What do you need for success?" instead of "What went wrong?"*

4. Utilize evidence-based practice. Processes must incorporate established patient-centered care guidelines and associated processes. Patient-centered care processes provide a structured approach to patient treatment plans, helping to reduce variability in care.

    * Remember that evidence-based practice is not static and may vary with circumstance.

5. Align resources and information at the point of care to optimize team performance. Open communication, feedback, and transparency are essential.

6. Make education and training a priority. Prioritizing and providing health workers with additional training and resources will increase their understanding of patient care needs, leading to more informed decisions about patient treatment processes.

    * Educate and train healthcare professionals to use all available resources, including tools like checklists and technology.

7. Provide actionable, accurate information.

   * Utilizing data analytics allows healthcare providers to make the best patient care decisions and to adapt to variability. Advanced analytics, including AI, can optimize decision-making by incorporating patient factors like age, gender, and medical history.

8. Leverage technology.

   * Automate and streamline aspects of patient care processes to improve accuracy by removing potential human error from critical decision-making steps.

9. Create an environment where everyone contributes to high-quality patient care.

   * Reward innovation and transformative change. Creating accountability systems for healthcare professionals helps ensure that patient care processes are performed consistently and accurately. Optimize processes by understanding how each step contributes to patient outcomes. Develop and continually improve reliable processes focused on patient safety and quality.

   * Monitor patient outcomes. Ongoing monitoring of patient outcomes will help healthcare providers identify trends in patient care and make necessary changes as needed.

10. Be compassionate.

ACKNOWLEDGMENTS

My motivation for writing this book came from two sources. First, the many patients I have been fortunate to care for and to be a part of their lives. Over the years, I heard so many stories of challenges and sometimes negative experiences people had navigating the health system no matter where in the world they lived. Similarly, I listened as physicians, nurses, and other caregivers expressed frustration when faced with rigid policies and processes that conflicted with what they believed was necessary to provide the best patient care. As I began to help teams with process improvement projects and saw success in improving patient care, people would tell me, "You should write a book." Finally, I took their advice to heart, and *The Process Manifesto* is the result.

There are, consequently, many people I have been privileged to meet and work with and care for around the world who deserve my deepest gratitude. This book is dedicated to the patient in every one of us who deserves effective, safe, and compassionate care.

I must also thank everyone I worked with on Steve Harrison's team. They helped me turn my thoughts and writing into this book. Cristina, Valerie, Christy, and Steve all motivated me to express my passion for doing the right thing for patients into a form that I hope will inspire others to improve processes that, in turn, improves access to care and the health of others.

I want to extend a special thanks to Dr. James Doty, who graciously offered to write the foreword. His commitment to compassion and understanding the needs of others has made an impression on me that has helped me think about process improvement from the human perspective, avoiding the trap of seeing process as a purely mechanical exercise.

Finally, I owe everything to my family, especially my wife Jeanette, who has always supported my commitment to improving things and not accepting the status quo, even when those presented challenges. I thank my parents for encouraging me to pursue a medical career from a very early age. Last but definitely not least, my children, Lauren, Christina, and Austin, who are amazing people and have taught me humility and kindness.

ENDNOTES

Prologue

1. Davidson I, Gallieni M, Saxena R, Dolmatch B. A patient centered decision-making dialysis access algorithm. J Vasc Access. 2007 Apr-Jun;8(2):59-68

Introduction

2. https://healthsystemsfacts.org/?gad=1&gclid=Cj0KCQjw5f2lBhCkARIsA-HeTvlhfrPs2jWJPkXgegWMmSpLPfydKI8OGF0-KAAnrwhlQF9HH-hw928YgaAtJdEALw_wcB/ (2023)

Chapter 1

3. W. Edwards Deming 2012. The Essential Deming: Leadership Principles from the Father of Total Quality Management. McGraw Hill.
4. K. Scott Griffith 2023. The Leader's Guide to Managing Risk: A Proven Method to Build Resilience and Reliability. HarperCollins.
5. Makary MA, Daniel M. Medical error-the third leading cause of death in the US. BMJ. 2016 May 3;353:i2139. doi: 10.1136/bmj.i2139. PMID: 27143499.
6. American Health Information Management Association (AHIMA). Process Flow Improvement: Principles, Methods, and Tools. AHIMA; 2014. Available at https://library.ahima.org/doc?oid=301597&fmt=pdf&pid=#page=33&view=fitH900V600 / (2023) and Centers for Medicare and Medicaid Services. Implementing Process Flow Improvements: A Guide to Quality Improvement Strategies. CMS; 2009. Available at https://www.cms.gov/Outreach-and-Education/Medicare-Learning-NetworkMLNProducts/downloads/implement_processflow_improvements_guidepdf.pdf?bhcp=1&utm_source=silverchair&utm_medium=email&utm_campaign=article_alert-jamanetworkopen&utm_content=olf&utm_term=07032020 / (2023)

Chapter 2

7. Liker, Jeffrey K. 2004. The Toyota Way: 14 Management Principles from the World's Greatest Manufacturer. New York: McGraw-Hill.
8. Majchrzak, Ann & Wang, Qianwei. Breaking the Functional Mind-Set in Process Organizations. Harvard Business Review 1996; Sept-Oct:93-99.

9. Duff, Sacha & Windham, T. & Wiegmann, Douglas & Kring, Jason & Schaus, Jennifer & Malony, Robert & Boquet, Albert. (2010). Identification and Classification of Flow Disruptions in the Operating Room during Two Types of General Surgery Procedures. Proceedings of the Human Factors and Ergonomics Society Annual Meeting. 54. 884-888. 10.1177/154193121005401217 and Slakey, D. P., Sargut, G., Glowacki, N. E., Katoozian, P. Y., Baylis, W. J., & Anderson, E. J. (2022). Using Process Flow Disruption Analysis to Guide Quality Improvement. *Journal of the American College of Surgeons*, 234(4), 557–564. https://doi.org/10.1097/XCS.0000000000000097

10. Slakey DP, George JS, Anderson E, Willeumier D, Guglielmi K. Applying international organization for standards 9001 to create an effective surgical quality committee. Am J Surg. 2021 Mar;221(3):598-601. doi: 10.1016/j.amjsurg.2020.11.014. Epub 2020 Nov 9. PMID: 33189310.

Chapter 3

11. https://www.airlines.org/impact / (2023)
12. Fujita S, Iida S, Nagai Y, Shimamori Y, Koyano K, Moriyama Y, Hasegawa T. Estimation of the number of patient deaths recognized by a medical practitioner as caused by adverse events in hospitals in Japan: A cross-sectional study. Medicine (Baltimore). 2017 Sep;96(39):e8128. doi: 10.1097/MD.0000000000008128. PMID: 28953645; PMCID: PMC5626288.
13. Excerpt from the 'Special Message to the Congress on Urgent National Needs'. NASA. May 24, 2004. https://www.nasa.gov/vision/space/features/jfk_speech_text.html / (2023).
14. Sargut G, McGrath RG. Learning to live with complexity. Harv Bus Rev 2011;89:68-76, 136.

Chapter 4

15. Gawande, Atul. 2011. *The Checklist Manifesto*. London, England: Profile Books.
16. Haynes, A. B., Weiser, T. G., Berry, W. R., Lipsitz, S. R., Breizat, A. H., Dellinger, E. P., Herbosa, T., Joseph, S., Kibatala, P. L., Lapitan, M. C., Merry, A. F., Moorthy, K., Reznick, R. K., Taylor, B., Gawande, A. A., & Safe Surgery Saves Lives Study Group (2009). A surgical safety checklist to reduce morbidity and mortality in a global population. *The New England Journal of Medicine*, 360(5), 491–499. https://doi.org/10.1056/NEJMsa0810119
17. Checklists to Improve Patient Safety, American Hospital Association, https://www.aha.org/ahahret-guides/2013-07-10-checklists-improve-patient-safe-

ty / (2023) and Checklists. Agency for Healthcare Research and Quality (AHRQ), 2019. https://psnet.ahrq.gov/primer/checklists / (2023) and Thomassen, Ø., Espeland, A., Søfteland, E. *et al.* Implementation of checklists in health care; learning from high-reliability organizations. *Scand J Trauma Resusc Emerg Med* 19, 53 (2011). https://doi.org/10.1186/1757-7241-19-53

18. Salas, E., Wilson, K. A., Burke, C. S., Wightman, D. C., & Howse, W. R. (2006). A Checklist for Crew Resource Management Training. Ergonomics in Design, 14(2), 6–15. https://doi.org/10.1177/106480460601400204 and https://www.visavi.com/articles/what-is-situational-awareness-and-why-is-it-so-relevant-for-industrial-operations?hsLang=en /(2023).

19. Thomassen Ø, Espeland A, Søfteland E, Lossius HM, Heltne JK, Brattebø G. Implementation of checklists in health care; learning from high-reliability organizations. Scand J Trauma Resusc Emerg Med. 2011 Oct 3;19:53. doi: 10.1186/1757-7241-19-53. PMID: 21967747; PMCID: PMC3205016. Clay-Williams R, Colligan L. Back to basics: checklists in aviation and health-care. *BMJ Quality & Safety* 2015;24:428-431.

Chapter 5

20. Kelly, Yvelynne & Mendu, Mallika. (2019). Breaking down health care silos. Harvard business review. https://hbr.org/2019/07/breaking-down-health-care-silos

21. Garstka ME, Slakey DP, Martin CA, Simms ER, Korndorffer JR Jr. Effectiveness of systems changes suggested by simulation of adverse surgical outcomes. BMJ Simul Technol Enhanc Learn. 2015 Dec 1;1(3):83-86. doi: 10.1136/bmjstel-2015-000055. PMID: 35515203; PMCID: PMC8990181.

22. Slakey DP, Davidson I. Surgeons lead educational program to improve kidney care in Vietnam. Bull Am Coll Surg. 2013 Oct;98(10):34-40. PMID: 24266117 and Douglas P. Slakey, Robert Reily, Ingemar Davidson, James R. Korndorffer. Evaluating a surgeon led training program: Targeting kidney disease in Vietnam. International Journal of Surgery Open. 2016 (Volume 4):18-22.

23. McChrystal, David Silverman, Tantum Collins, Chris Fussell 2015. Team of Teams: New Rules of Engagement for a Complex World. General Stanley. Penguin Books Limited.

24. Katie Kaney 2023. Both/And: Medicine & Public Health Together. Telemachus Press, LLC.

25. Lorenz, EN. Deterministic nonperiodic flow. J Atmosph Sci 1963; 20:130-141.

26. Reeder-Hayes KE, Anderson BO. Breast Cancer Disparities at Home and Abroad: A Review of the Challenges and Opportunities for System-Level

Change. Clin Cancer Res. 2017 Jun 1;23(11):2655-2664. doi: 10.1158/1078-0432.CCR-16-2630. PMID: 28572260; PMCID: PMC5499686.

Chapter 6

27. W. Edwards Deming 2012. The Essential Deming: Leadership Principles from the Father of Total Quality Management. McGraw Hill.
28. https://www.uipath.com/blog/automation/ai-rpa-differences-when-to-use-them-together /(2023).
29. Simms ER, Slakey DP, Garstka ME, Tersigni SA, Korndorffer JR. Can simulation improve the traditional method of root cause analysis: a preliminary investigation. Surgery. 2012 Sep;152(3):489-97. doi: 10.1016/j.surg.2012.07.029. PMID: 22938908.
30. Slakey, D. P., Sargut, G., Glowacki, N. E., Katoozian, P. Y., Baylis, W. J., & Anderson, E. J. (2022). Using Process Flow Disruption Analysis to Guide Quality Improvement. *Journal of the American College of Surgeons*, 234(4), 557–564. https://doi.org/10.1097/XCS.0000000000000097
31. The Art of Service – Deming PDCA Publishing 2020. Deming PDCA A Complete Guide.
32. James, B. C., & Poulsen, G. P. (2016). The Case for Capitation. *Harvard business review*, 94(7-8), 102–134.

Chapter 7

33. Boeing Systems Approach – Risk Management Solutions for Aerospace. (2020). https://www.boeing.com/commercial/aeromagazine/articles/qtr_2_06/article_02_1.html. /(2023) and K. Scott Griffith 2023. The Leader's Guide to Managing Risk: A Proven Method to Build Resilience and Reliability. HarperCollins.
34. De Hert S. Burnout in Healthcare Workers: Prevalence, Impact and Preventative Strategies. Local Reg Anesth. 2020 Oct 28;13:171-183. doi: 10.2147/LRA.S240564. PMID: 33149664; PMCID: PMC7604257.
35. https://www.ahrq.gov/prevention/clinician/ahrq-works/burnout/index.html /(2023).
36. Rehder, K. J., Adair, K. C., Hadley, A., McKittrick, K., Frankel, A., Leonard, M., Frankel, T. C., & Sexton, J. B. (2020). Associations Between a New Disruptive Behaviors Scale and Teamwork, Patient Safety, Work-Life Balance, Burnout, and Depression. *The Joint Commission Journal on Quality and Patient Safety*, 46(1), 18-26. https://doi.org/10.1016/j.jcjq.2019.09.004

Chapter 8

37. Taurchini M, Del Naja C, Tancredi A. Enhanced Recovery After Surgery:a patient centered process. J Vis Surg. 2018 Feb 27;4:40. doi: 10.21037/jovs.2018.01.20. PMID: 29552522; PMCID: PMC5847857.

38. Kehlet, H., & Holte, K. (2001). Effect of postoperative analgesia on surgical outcome. *BJA: British Journal of Anaesthesia, 87(1), 62-72. https://doi.org/10.1093/bja/87.1.62*

39. Vandepitte C, Van Pachtenbeke L, Van Herreweghe I, Gupta RK, Elkassabany NM. Same Day Joint Replacement Surgery: Patient Selection and Perioperative Management. Anesthesiol Clin. 2022 Sep;40(3):537-545. doi: 10.1016/j.anclin.2022.04.003. Epub 2022 Jul 12. PMID: 36049880.

40. Cook DA, Pencille LJ, Dupras DM, Linderbaum JA, Pankratz VS, Wilkinson JM. Practice variation and practice guidelines: Attitudes of generalist and specialist physicians, nurse practitioners, and physician assistants. PLoS One. 2018 Jan 31;13(1):e0191943. doi: 10.1371/journal.pone.0191943. PMID: 29385203; PMCID: PMC5792011 and Gutacker N, Bloor K, Bojke C, Walshe K. Should interventions to reduce variation in care quality target doctors or hospitals? Health Policy. 2018 Jun;122(6):660-666. doi: 10.1016/j.healthpol.2018.04.004. Epub 2018 Apr 13. PMID: 29703654; PMCID: PMC6022214.

41. Porter, ME and Lee, TH. The strategy that will fix healthcare. HBR 2013 Oct;91910):50-70.

42. Gawande, A., et al. Effectiveness of a standardized protocol for postoperative care on 30-day mortality after major surgery. Health Affairs 2016;35(8): 1389–1396.

Chapter 9

43. Stephen Trzeciak, Anthony Mazzarelli, and Emma Seppälä. Leading with Compassion Has Research-Backed Benefits. Harvard Business Review. February 27, 2023

44. Jemal K, Hailu D, Mekonnen M, Tesfa B, Bekele K, Kinati T. The importance of compassion and respectful care for the health workforce: a mixed-methods study. Z Gesundh Wiss. 2023;31(2):167-178. doi: 10.1007/s10389-021-01495-0. Epub 2021 Mar 11. PMID: 33728258; PMCID: PMC7951938.

ADDITIONAL RESOURCES

Bias

Patiño-Alonso MC et al (2018). Impact of Heuristic Reasoning and Confirmation Bias on Clinical Decision Making: A Systematic Review. Journal of Educational Evaluation for Health Professions 15:15 doi: 10.3352/jeehp.2018.15.15

Marewski JN, Gigerenzer G. Heuristic decision making in medicine. Dialogues Clin Neurosci. 2012 Mar;14(1):77-89. doi: 10.31887/DCNS.2012.14.1/jmarewski. PMID: 22577307; PMCID: PMC3341653.

Tversky, Amos, and Daniel Kahneman. "Judgment under Uncertainty: Heuristics and Biases." *Science* 185, no. 4157 (1974): 1124–31.

Checklists

Anderson R & Bostrom A (2019). How checklists can improve patient safety, quality of care and reduce costs in healthcare organizations: a review of the literature and recommendations for implementation strategies. BMC Health Services Research 19(1):76 doi:10.1186/s12913-019-3972-9

Scott TJ (2019). The Utility of Checklists for Enhancing Safety Culture and Quality Improvement in Healthcare Organizations: A Review of the Literature, Medical Education Online 24(1):1574355 doi: 10.1080/10872981.2019.1574355.

Spiliopoulou A et al (2019). Barriers to checklists use in healthcare settings: a systematic review and qualitative synthesis of the literature. BMC Health Services Research 19(1):705 doi:10.1186/s12913-019-4485-0

"Checklists and Their Role in Airline Safety". Skybrary Aviation Safety. 2019. https://skybrary.aero/index.php/Checklists_and_Their_Role_in_Airline_Safety

"The Benefits of Crew Resource Management". Airways Magazine, July 2016. https://www.airwaysmag.com/flightcrew/benefits-crew-resource-management/

"Checklist: What the Law Requires". FAA Safety Briefing. 2018. https://www.faasafetybriefing.com/2018/09/checklist-what-law-requires/.

Information

"Healthcare Analytics: What It Is & How Data Analysis Improves Care Delivery" – Health Catalyst (2020) https://www.healthcatalyst.com/what-is-healthcare-analytics

"The Role of Artificial Intelligence in Healthcare" – Yottamine Analytics (2018) https://www.yottamine.com/blog/the-role-of-artificial-intelligence-in-healthcare

"Using patient analytics to improve patient experience and outcomes" – McKinsey (2019) https://www.mckinsey.com/industries/health-care-systems-and-services/our-insights/using-patientanalytics to improve patient experience and outcomes.

Health Catalyst (2020) "Healthcare Analytics: What It Is & How Data Analysis Improves Care Delivery" https://www.healthcatalyst.com/what-is-healthcare-analytics

Process Flow

American Medical Association. Enhancing Patient Safety through Process Flow Redesign and Technology Integration in Health Care. 2009. Available at https://www.ama-assn.org/delivering-care/patient-safety/enhancing-patient-safety-through process flow redesign and technology integration in healthcare

Schmitt MH, et al. Process Flow Improvement: A Multifaceted Approach to Reduce Unnecessary Healthcare Costs and Improve Quality of Care. JAMA Network Open; 2019. Availablehttps://jamanetwork.com/journals/jamanetworkopen/fullarticle/2729066?utm_source=Silverchair&utm_medium=email&utm_campaign=article_alert-jamanetworkopen&utm_content=olf&utm_term=07032020

Reliability

Hollnagel, E., Woods, D., & Leveson, N. (2009). Resilience engineering concepts and precepts. Farnham ; Burlington : Ashgate Pub. Ltd. doi:10.1007/s00500-014-1466-3.

Ramos-Munoz, J., & Vostal, F. (2018). Lean Six Sigma in healthcare and patient safety: A systematic review. International Journal of Quality & Reliability Management, 35(7), 1298–1321. doi:10.1108/ijqrm-02-2017-0039

Hollnagel, E., Woods, D., & Leveson, N. (2009). Resilience engineering concepts and precepts. Farnham ; Burlington : Ashgate Pub. Ltd. doi:10.1007/s00500-014-1466-3.

Leveson, N., & Turner, C. S .(2018). A New Accident Model for Engineering Safer Systems: Resilience Engineering for High Reliability Organizations . IEEE Aerospace and Electronic Systems Magazine, 33(2), 3–13. doi:10.1109/maes.2018.2791957.

Gummesson, E., Högberg, P., & Forsman, M.(2010). Applying patient safety research to the lean production system — implications for patient safety improvement strategies: a descriptive case study from Sweden's leading university hospital. Quality Management in Health Care, 19(2), 109–118. doi:10.1097/qmh.0b013e3181cdc8a7.

Antonacci, L., & Cerulli, C.(2017). Lean Six Sigma in healthcare: A systematic review of the literature (2005-2016). International Journal of Quality & Reliability Management ,34(6/7), 871–896. doi:10.1108/ijqrm-02-2015-0028.

Systems

Carey, E., Sharma, R., Colleran, K., and Lyle, D.(2014). Opportunities for patient safety improvement through application of complexity science principles in the operating room . BMJ Quality & Safety , 23(4), 256–263. doi:10.1136/bmjqs-2013-002032.

Rugh, Wilson J 1981. Nonlinear System Theory: The Volterra / Wiener Approach. The Johns Hopkins University Press.

Thurner, Stefan, Peter Klimek, and Rudolf Hanel, **Introduction to the Theory of Complex Systems** (Oxford, 2018; online edn, Oxford Academic, 22 Nov. 2018), https://doi.org/10.1093/oso/9780198821939.001.0001, accessed 30 Mar. 2023.

Heinrichs-Kreutzer, S., Sieckmann, C., & Loebell, A. (2018). The Influence of Complexity Thinking on Innovation Performance—A Study Based on the Aerospace Industry. Sustainability, 10(10), 3576. doi:10.3390/su10103576

Eppich WJ, Arora S, Howard SK et al (2013) A framework for patient safety in complex healthcare systems . BMJ Qual Saf 22: i33–i41 . doi:10.1136/bmjqs-2012-001083

Kaplan, G., G. Bo-Linn, P. Carayon, P. Pronovost, W. Rouse, P. Reid, and R. Saunders. 2013. Bringing a Systems Approach to Health. *NAM Perspectives*. Discussion Paper, National Academy of Medicine, Washington, DC. https://doi.org/10.31478/201307a

Value

Hendrickx T, Kessous L (2015) The patient as the center of a value based health care system. J Eval Clin Pract 21: 277–282 . doi:10.1111/jep.12358

Neuhauser D, Riley RD (2009) What is patient safety culture? A review of the literature and recommendations for further development of the science. Qual Saf Health Care 18: 29–35 . doi:10.1136/qshc.2008.029497

Better Patient Flow Means Breaking Down the Silos. Institute for Healthcare Improvement. https://www.ihi.org/resources/Pages/ImprovementStories/BetterPatientFlowMeansBreakingDowntheSilos.aspx

Shrank WH, Rogstad TL, Parekh N. Waste in the US Health Care System: Estimated Costs and Potential for Savings. *JAMA*. 2019;322(15):1501–1509. doi:10.1001/jama.2019.13978

Womack, J., & Jones, D. (2005). Lean Thinking : Banish Waste and Create Wealth in Your Corporation , Revised and Updated . New York : Simon & Schuster Paperbacks ; London : Profile Books Ltd.. ISBN-13: 9780743249275.

Bentley TG, Effros RM, Palar K, Keeler EB. Waste in the U.S. Health care system: a conceptual framework. Milbank Q. 2008 Dec;86(4):629-59. doi: 10.1111/j.1468-0009.2008.00537.x. PMID: 19120983; PMCID: PMC2690367.

Bauchner, H., & Fontanarosa, P. B. (2019). Waste in the US Health Care System. *JAMA*, 322(15), 1463–1464. https://doi.org/10.1001/jama.2019.15353

ABOUT THE AUTHOR

DR. DOUGLAS SLAKEY is an internationally recognized transplant surgeon, educator, healthcare professional, and administrator. Doug is currently a professor of surgery at the University of Illinois, Chicago, and the president of Process Health Consulting, a healthcare consultancy focused on enhancing and optimizing operations and process flow, emphasizing complex system management strategies that optimize patient outcomes. He is a global educator, consultant, author, and speaker who inspires healthcare teams to provide effective, compassionate patient care.

Made in the USA
Middletown, DE
04 September 2024

59793774R00106